Comments from readers on *Type 2 Diabetes: Answers at your fingertips*:

'I can pass on much more information now after this marathon read! I'll be the first to purchase the new edition when it's published.'

CLARE MEHMET,
Diabetes UK Newham Voluntary Group

'It is an invaluable guide to the subject: authoritative, nicely written and packed with facts.'

P L,
Acton

'This book will go a long way in helping anyone diagnosed with diabetes – or their relatives – understand what lies ahead. It explains everything you need to know about what causes diabetes and how to manage it.'

JIMMY TARBUCK,
Honorary Vice-President Diabetes UK

Comments on earlier editions from readers

'An excellent book. It is comprehensive, informative, and easy to read and understand.'

DON KENDRICK,
Seaton, Devon

'A marvellous book – just what the layman needs.'

MRS P PILLEY,
Hornchurch

'I like the form it takes (questions and answers); it makes it much easier to find the specific areas when a problem does arise. Also it makes easier reading for picking up and putting down without having to wade through chapter after chapter of heavy medical jargon which for the lay person can be very difficult to take in and understand.'

MRS PAM MUNFORD,
Lincoln

'I have read the book myself from cover to cover and found it to be most informative, up-to-date and presented in a format which is easy to assimilate by the majority of people with diabetes who will undoubtedly relate some question to a particular experience of their own – and find the answer.'

PHILIP WHITMORE,
Macclesfield

'I think the book is excellent value since it answers all the basic questions of diabetes and has answers to questions I have not seen written down before. (In fact the whole family is interested in reading it.)'

D BALL,
Nottingham

Reviews of previous editions

'Overall this is a most interesting and useful book suitable for people with diabetes, their families, health professionals and anyone interested in diabetes. It is a book that once bought will be used over and over again, and works out to be good value.'

BALANCE

'... a guide, in lively question and answer form, to coping with diabetes. It is quite possible to lead a full life providing the sufferer understands and can control the disease.'

WOMAN'S JOURNAL

'Has positive information to help both young and old lead active lives with the minimum of restrictions.'

GOOD HOUSEKEEPING

'I would recommend it to people living with diabetes, but also to professionals in the diabetes field.'

PROFESSIONAL NURSE

'The book is well presented, with good, clear illustrations and is reasonably priced. I highly recommend it for people newly diagnosed with diabetes and their families and as a source of reference for nurses dealing with diabetes.'

NURSING STANDARD

'Woe betide any clinicians or nurses whose patients have read this invaluable source of down-to-earth information when they have not.'

THE LANCET

'The book's ultimate merit is that it answers all the basic questions around diabetes while being a continuing resource to manage real-life events as they occur.'

DIABETIC MEDICINE

This seventh edition is dedicated to Peter Sönksen and Sue Judd whose inspiration and energy led to the first edition of the book.

Type 2 Diabetes

Answers at your fingertips

SEVENTH EDITION

Type 2 Diabetes

Answers at your fingertips

SEVENTH EDITION

Charles Fox BM, FRCP

*Consultant Physician with
Special Interest in Diabetes,
Northampton General Hospital*

Anne Kilvert MD, FRCP

*Consultant Physician with
Special Interest in Diabetes,
Northampton General Hospital*

Diabetes UK
The charity for
people with diabetes
is pleased to have worked
with Class Publishing
on this book

CLASS PUBLISHING · LONDON

Printing history
First published as *Diabetes at Your Fingertips* 1985; Reprinted 1987
Second edition, revised and expanded 1991; Reprinted with revisions 1991;
    Reprinted with revisions 1992
Third edition, revised and expanded 1994; Reprinted 1995, 1996;
    Reprinted with revisions 1997
Fourth edition, revised and expanded 1998; Reprinted with revisions 1999;
    Reprinted with revisions 2001; Reprinted 2002
Fifth edition 2003; Reprinted 2003; Reprinted 2004;
    Reprinted with revisions 2005; Reprinted 2006
Sixth edition (as two books, *Type 1 Diabetes* and *Type 2 Diabetes*) 2007
Seventh edition 2011

The authors and publishers welcome feedback from the users of this book. Please contact the publishers.
Class Health, The Exchange, Express Park,
Bristol Road, Bridgwater, TA6 4RR, UK
Telephone: 020 7371 2119   Fax: 020 7371 2878 [International +4420]
email: post@class.co.uk   Website: www.class.co.uk

A CIP catalogue for this book is available from the British Library

ISBN 978 1 85959 3 233

10 9 8 7 6 5 4 3 2 1

Edited by Wendy Mould

Cartoons by Jane Taylor

Line illustrations by David Woodroffe

Designed by Martin Bristow

Typeset by Mach 3 Solutions Ltd

Printed and bound in Great Britain by the MPG Books Group

Contents

Foreword *by Sir Steve Redgrave* CBE   xi

Foreword to the 6th edition *by Peter Sönksen and Sue Judd*   xii

Preface   xiii

Acknowledgements   xiv

Introduction   xv

1 What is diabetes?   1

What happens in diabetes?   2

Types of diabetes   5

Causes of diabetes   7

Symptoms   21

2 Treatment without insulin   24

Diabetes education   25

Diet   27

Exercise   47

Tablets   50

Injections other than insulin   60

Non-medical treatments   62

3 Treatment with insulin 65

Types of insulin 66

Timing 77

Dosage 81

Injecting 83

Diet and insulin 91

Hypos 101

4 Monitoring and control 107

Why monitor? 109

Monitoring in Type 2 diabetes 112

Blood glucose testing 113

Urine 126

Haemoglobin A$_{1c}$ 129

Diabetes clinics 133

5 Life with diabetes 146

Sports 147

Eating out 150

Fasting and diabetes 150

Holidays and travel 151

Work 160

Other illnesses 164

Hospital operations 168

Driving 170

Alcohol 175

Drugs   177

Smoking   179

Prescription charges and Social Security benefits   181

Miscellaneous   183

6 Sex, contraception and HRT   187

Impotence (Erectile dysfunction)   188

Contraception and vasectomy   194

Thrush   197

Hormone Replacement Therapy (HRT)   198

Termination of pregnancy   200

Fertility   200

7 Pregnancy   202

Prepregnancy   204

Pregnancy management   208

Complications   211

8 Long-term complications   217

General questions   219

Eyes   223

Feet, podiatry and footwear   231

Kidney damage   242

Nerve damage   245

Heart and blood vessel disease   249

Blood pressure   253

The mind   254

9 Research and the future   256

Searching for causes and cures   257
Transplantation   258
New treatments   260
Possible developments in insulin delivery   261
Insulin pumps and artificial pancreas   263

10 Self-help groups   266

Diabetes UK   266
Juvenile Diabetes Research Foundation (JDRF)   269
Insulin-Pumpers   269
Insulin Dependent Diabetes Trust (IDDT)   270
National Kidney Federation (NKF)   270

11 Emergencies   272

Glossary   279

Appendix 1: Publications   290

Appendix 2: Useful addresses   292

Index   299

Foreword

by **Sir Steve Redgrave** CBE
Vice-President, Diabetes UK

Diabetes: Answers at your fingertips has always – in its six editions, published over 20 years – shown a very constructive and positive approach to dealing with diabetes. Its layout encourages readers to develop a good understanding of their condition and to question their approach to the disease.

This new seventh edition maintains the same positive approach, and is now in two parallel versions: one specifically for people with Type 1 diabetes, the other written for people with Type 2 diabetes.

I have no hesitation in commending this book, which helps towards our understanding of diabetes as well as being very constructive in dealing with issues that surround the condition. I have always maintained that 'I have diabetes but it doesn't have me.' As well as going out and leading a very active and normal life, not allowing diabetes to restrain you in any way, learning more about diabetes is also very positive. Happy reading.

Foreword to the 6th edition

Peter Sönksen and Sue Judd
Co-authors of previous editions

After 20 years with *Diabetes at your fingertips*, we were delighted to read this new book and to be invited to write a Foreword. Sensibly, the authors and publishers have decided that it would now be better to have two versions designed specifically for Type 1 and 2 diabetes.

There is a global pandemic of Type 2 diabetes, and this book will be of great value to all these people, as well as to any of their friends and family who wish to explore the condition and its treatment in more detail. It will also be invaluable to the professional medical and paramedical staff responsible for delivering care to people with diabetes, particularly those in the community.

Written in the now familiar 'questions and answers' format, it is designed for dipping into rather than cover-to-cover reading, but newly diagnosed patients might well like to read its contents *in toto* and will benefit from doing so.

The secret to successful self-care is knowledge, confidence and motivation; this new book will make a significant, positive contribution to this important area.

Peter Sönksen MD, FRCP, FFSEM (UK)
Emeritus Professor of Endocrinology

Sue Judd SRN
*Retired Diabetes Specialist Nurse
St Thomas' Hospital, London*

Preface

Is this the right book for you? Do you have Type 2 diabetes?

This is the seventh edition of *Diabetes: answers at your fingertips* and in the sixth edition we made some important changes which have been expanded upon. The original book was designed to answer questions about both Type 1 and Type 2 diabetes. In the new version, we have decided to write separate books for Type 1 and Type 2 diabetes and this book is for people with Type 2 diabetes.

You may not be sure which type of diabetes you have. There is a general rule that people with Type 1 diabetes are usually young, tend to be underweight at the time of diagnosis and need treatment with insulin straight away. People with Type 2 diabetes are more likely to be overweight when diagnosed and are usually over 30. They can be treated with diet and tablets and do not often need insulin in the early years, although they may do so later.

Unfortunately Type 2 diabetes is becoming an increasing problem in children's clinics and in some parts of USA half the children have type 2 diabetes. This book addresses the particular problems of type 2 diabetes in young people.

If your diabetes has been successfully treated at the onset with diet or tablets or both, this book is for you.

Acknowledgements

We are grateful to all the people who helped in the production of past editions of *Diabetes at your fingertips*: Anna Fox, Peter Swift, Clara Lowy, Suzanne Lucas and Judith North.

Peter Sönksen and Sue Judd had the original idea of a question and answer book for people with diabetes (*The Diabetes Reference Book*). This new edition is based on their text and the clear practical advice they gave.

We thank the following writers for their contributions to the new edition: Florence Brown for providing the nursing perspective in the chapters on insulin and monitoring; Helen Millar for answers to the questions on diet; and Maria Mousley for the podiatry section.

We would like to thank the people who reviewed the book and provided helpful advice: Peter Sönksen and Sue Judd, Vasso Vydelingum for a cultural perspective, Peter Lapsley, Claire Mehmet and finally Rosie Walker for a detailed critique.

Our editors Caroline Sheldrick, Richenda Milton-Daws and Wendy Mould have been both encouraging and endlessly patient. Jane Taylor drew the new cartoons. Richard Warner of Class Publishing has been the driving force.

Introduction

If you are reading this, you or someone you know may well have been found to have Type 2 diabetes. Although more and more people are developing this condition, it is often discovered by chance either during a routine medical check-up or following a serious medical condition such as a heart attack.

Two problems come together to cause Type 2 diabetes. First, there is a failure to produce enough insulin, and second, there is resistance in the body to the action of this insulin, which is most commonly related to obesity. Many populations have seen a rise in body weight and a decrease in exercise as a result of changes in lifestyle, and this is responsible for the massive global increase in Type 2 diabetes.

Diabetes may be present for months or even years before it is discovered, and during this time silent damage may be done to vulnerable parts of the body such as the eyes, heart, kidneys and feet. Efforts are being made to diagnose diabetes at an early stage so that treatment can be introduced to protect people from these complications.

Once detected, Type 2 diabetes can usually be treated with diet and tablets at first, but the condition progresses with time and most people will eventually need insulin. Unfortunately there is no cure for diabetes but treatment can keep people healthy, especially if they can learn to take diabetes in their stride.

We hope this book will help you understand Type 2 diabetes and give you the information you need.

HOW TO USE THIS BOOK

Most chapters comprise a series of questions and answers, and are not designed to be read from beginning to end. However, some chapters could well be read through at the outset, in particular Chapter 1: **What is diabetes?**, Chapter 4: **Monitoring and control**, and Chapter 8: **Long-term complications**.

If you are newly diagnosed, you may not be ready to come to grips with Chapter 9: **Research and the future** but you may want to discover what is known about the causes of diabetes (in Chapter 1). If you have just started insulin injections you should read the following sections at an early stage.

- Hypos (in Chapter 3)

- Other illnesses (in Chapter 5)

- Types of insulin (in Chapter 3)

- Monitoring in Type 2 diabetes (in Chapter 4)

- Blood glucose testing (in Chapter 4)

- Driving (in Chapter 5)

- Emergencies (Chapter 11)

More experienced people will want to test us out in Chapter 5: **Life with diabetes** to see if our answers coincide with their own experience.

There is bound to be some repetition in a book of this sort, but we think it is better to deal with similar topics under separate headings rather than ask the reader to shuffle from one end of the book to the other. We have tried to be consistent in our answers.

Feedback is the most important feature of good diabetes care. This relies on people being honest with the doctor or nurse and vice versa. Not everyone will agree with the answers we give, but the book can only be improved if you let us know when you disagree and have found our advice to be unhelpful. We would also like to know if there are important questions that we have not covered. Please write to us c/o Class Publishing, Barb House, Barb Mews, London W6 7PA, UK or email post@class.co.uk.

1 | What is diabetes?

In this chapter we describe the central problem in diabetes, which is an increase in the amount of glucose (sugar) in the blood. We explain why this happens and why it may be dangerous.

There are two main types of diabetes:

- Type 1 – this type of diabetes usually appears in younger people under the age of 40 but may occur at any age. It is treated by insulin injections and diet;

- Type 2 – this type of diabetes usually appears in people over the age of 40 but is becoming more common in younger age groups as a result of the increase in obesity in the general population. Type 2 diabetes may go undetected for many years and because people do not always feel unwell, it may be discovered by chance at a routine medical. It usually responds well to diet or tablets but as it is a progressive condition, most people need insulin treatment eventually.

There may be mild symptoms such as thirst, tiredness and passing excess urine, which should disappear once treatment is established. There are other rare types of diabetes, which we also mention in this chapter.

Diabetes is often detected following a routine blood or urine test for glucose and it may therefore exist for many years without being discovered. People in this situation often feel perfectly well at the time diabetes is diagnosed. Unfortunately, undetected diabetes may over a period of years lead to complications affecting eyes, nerves and blood vessels.

WHAT HAPPENS IN DIABETES?

The pancreas is a gland situated in the upper part of the abdomen and connected by a fine tube to the intestine (see Figure 1.1). One of its functions is to release into the gut digestive juices, which are mixed with food soon after it leaves the stomach.

These digestive juices are needed to break down food and help it be absorbed into the body. This part of the pancreas has nothing to do with diabetes.

The pancreas also produces a number of hormones which are released directly into the bloodstream, unlike the digestive juices which pass into the intestine. The most important of these hormones is insulin and a shortage of this causes diabetes. The other important hormone produced by the pancreas is glucagon, which has the opposite action to insulin and may be used in correcting serious hypos. ('Hypo' is short for hypoglycaemia, meaning low blood sugar. See the section *Hypos* in Chapter 3). Both hormones come from a part of the pancreas called the islets of Langerhans, which are scattered throughout the pancreas.

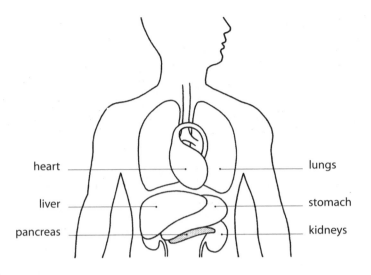

Figure 1.1 Location of the pancreas

Why does the body need insulin?

Without insulin the body cannot make use of the food we eat. Food is broken down in the stomach and intestine into simple chemicals, such as glucose and fatty acids, which provide fuel for all the activities of the body. These simple chemicals also provide building blocks for growth or replacing worn out parts, and any extra is stored for later use. In diabetes, food is broken down as normal but, because of the shortage of insulin (or sometimes because insulin does not work properly), excess glucose cannot be stored and builds up in the bloodstream. When glucose rises above a certain level, it spills into the urine through the kidneys.

The liver plays a dual role in processing food. It converts simple chemicals into complex substances which are then stored for future use and it also allows breakdown of these stores when they are needed for fuel. This process is controlled by insulin. For example, in the absence of insulin, glycogen (starch) is broken down into glucose, which pours out of the liver into the bloodstream (and then into the urine). Insulin

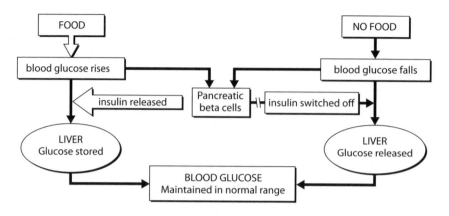

Figure 1.2 Insulin production system

switches off this outpouring of glucose and causes the glucose to be stored as glycogen. Thus insulin ensures that a perfect balance is kept between the production of glucose and its storage, and in this way it maintains the blood glucose at a normal level. Insulin plays other important roles, such as allowing glucose to get into other parts of the body to be used as a fuel, and regulating the processing of amino acids and fatty acids, which are the breakdown products of protein and fat.

What happens to insulin production in diabetes?

In people who do not have diabetes, insulin is produced in the pancreas and released into the blood as soon as the blood glucose level starts to rise after eating. Insulin travels straight from the pancreas to the liver where it has the important role of regulating glucose production and the storage of glucose as glycogen. The level of glucose in the blood then falls and, as it does so, insulin production is switched off, allowing glucose to be released from stores in the liver (see Figure 1.2). In people who do not have diabetes this sensitive system keeps the amount of glucose in the blood at a steady level.

In diabetes this process is faulty. People with Type 2 diabetes can still produce some insulin but not in adequate amounts to keep the blood glucose level normal. This is because their insulin does not work properly (a condition called 'insulin resistance'). People with Type 1 diabetes have little or no insulin of their own and need injections of insulin to try to keep the blood glucose level normal. Even if given four or five times a day, injected insulin is not as efficient at regulating blood glucose as the pancreas, which responds instantly to small changes in blood glucose by switching the insulin supply on or off.

There are three main factors affecting the level of glucose in the blood:

- food (which puts it up);
- insulin (which brings it down);
- exercise (which also brings it down).

Any form of stress, such as an illness like flu, increases blood glucose. Learning how to balance your blood glucose level in diabetes is a matter of trial and error. This involves taking a lot of blood glucose measurements and discovering how various foods and forms of exercise affect the levels.

TYPES OF DIABETES

I hadn't realised that there were different types of diabetes until I was diagnosed with what my GP called Type 2. What is the difference between my diabetes and Type 1 diabetes?

Diabetes does exist in different forms. Two main types are recognised.

- Type 1 diabetes usually occurs in younger people. This condition develops suddenly and insulin injections are nearly always needed as soon as it is diagnosed. About one in ten of all people with diabetes fall into this category, which used to be called 'insulin dependent diabetes'.

- Type 2 diabetes usually occurs in older people, who are often overweight, and have less obvious symptoms. Obesity is linked to insulin resistance, which is a root cause of Type 2 diabetes and insulin resistance occurs many years before diabetes itself begins. As the population becomes more overweight, Type 2 diabetes is developing in younger age groups, including children. At the onset of Type 2 diabetes, treatment is with diet with or without tablets. After a few years, people with Type 2 diabetes nearly always need to use insulin, because of the progressive nature of this condition.

I have been told that I have diabetes insipidus. Is this the same as the diabetes that my friend's elderly father has?

The only connection between diabetes insipidus and the more common form of diabetes (the full name of which is diabetes mellitus) is that people with both conditions pass large amounts of urine. Diabetes insipidus is a rare condition caused by an abnormality in the pituitary gland and not the pancreas. One disorder does not lead to the other, and diabetes insipidus does not carry the risk of long-term complications found in diabetes mellitus.

My wife has just given birth to a baby boy who weighed 4.3 kg (9 lb 4 oz) at birth. Apparently she may have had diabetes while she was pregnant. Is this likely to happen again if we have another baby?

Women who give birth to heavy babies (over 4 kg or 9 lb 4 oz) may have had a raised blood glucose level during pregnancy. This extra glucose crosses the placenta into the unborn baby, who responds by producing extra insulin of its own. The combination of excess glucose and excess insulin makes the unborn baby grow fat and bloated. After birth the baby is cut off from the high glucose input and then runs the risk of a low blood glucose level (hypoglycaemia).

Women who develop diabetes during pregnancy have a condition called 'gestational diabetes'. In most women, the diabetes goes away after delivery, but a small number of women continue to have diabetes. Once the problem has been identified, it is very likely to recur during subsequent pregnancies. Provided that glucose levels are kept within normal limits (insulin may be needed for this), the baby will be a normal weight and will not be at risk.

Women who have diabetes during pregnancy are more likely to develop Type 2 diabetes later in life (see Chapter 7: **Pregnancy**).

CAUSES OF DIABETES

Despite a vast amount of research throughout the world the cause of diabetes is not known. Some families carry an extra risk of diabetes (see the section *Inheritance* on p. 16).

Why have I got diabetes?

The short answer is that your pancreas is no longer making enough insulin for your body's needs. The long answer, as to why this has happened, is not so easy because the causes are not well understood – but there are a few clues. Diabetes often runs in families (see the section *Inheritance* on p. 16). Other possible causes are discussed in this section. It is not rare and in the UK, about three people in 100 are known to have diabetes and at least two in 100 have diabetes but don't know it – the so called 'missing million', publicised by Diabetes UK. About three children per 1000 have diabetes and the risk is increasing, particularly in young children below the age of 5 years.

Could diabetes be triggered by a virus?

Some scientists used to suspect that a certain virus could be the cause of diabetes in young people but proof is lacking and this theory now seems very unlikely to be true.

There is certainly no 'diabetes virus' and you cannot catch diabetes in the same way as chickenpox. There is no suggestion that Type 2 diabetes could be caused by a virus infection.

I was very overweight when I was diagnosed with diabetes. Can this have caused my diabetes?

If you have a genetic tendency towards diabetes, being over-weight may bring on the disease, particularly if you carry excess fat around the abdomen (central obesity). This stops insulin from lowering the blood sugar effectively, a condition known as 'insulin resistance', which is the underlying cause of Type 2 diabetes. With the worldwide increase in obesity, Type 2 diabetes is becoming increasingly common. In the past, it usually affected the middle-aged and elderly, but it is now common in a younger age group and is no longer unusual in children's clinics.

In most cases this type of diabetes can be controlled at first by diet and weight loss. Recent recommendations advise starting metformin tablets (see p. 53) as soon as the condition is diagnosed. Many people with diabetes who are overweight find it hard to lose weight; others find that strict dieting alone is not enough to lower the blood glucose and they have to take tablets, insulin injections or a combination of the two.

You will find more information about diet and diabetes and being overweight in Chapter 2.

I have just been diagnosed with Type 2 diabetes and my doctor says it is because I have something called the Metabolic Syndrome. What does this mean and is it the cause of my diabetes?

Metabolic syndrome is a group of conditions that are known to increase the risk of heart disease and stroke. There are a number of different definitions but they all emphasise that insulin resistance is the underlying cause. The cluster of problems called metabolic syndrome includes the following:

- central obesity (fat around the waist line)

- high blood pressure

- abnormal cholesterol (high LDL and low HDL fractions) and high levels of triglycerides

- Type 2 diabetes, impaired glucose tolerance (see link) – or at least a high risk of developing this

- fatty liver (see next question)

The insulin resistance means that if a person with metabolic syndrome does not have diabetes, their beta cells in the pancreas will be working overtime to produce high levels of insulin in order to keep the blood sugar level normal. There is a high chance that the beta cells will be unable to maintain this high output of insulin indefinitely and sooner or later the blood sugar level will rise, resulting in diabetes.

People with metabolic syndrome, whether or not they have diabetes, will probably be asked to take a number of tablets in order to correct the high blood pressure and abnormal cholesterol levels. The best treatment (though not always the easiest) is to reduce weight and overcome the central obesity.

My doctor carries out regular tests for diabetes. This is because I have a condition called fatty liver, which he says puts me at risk of developing diabetes in the future.

The medical name for this condition is Non-Alcoholic Fatty Liver Disease (NAFLD) and it describes a range of conditions in which the liver tests are abnormal in people who drink little or no alcohol. It ranges from a mild condition in which excess fat is deposited in the liver causing slightly abnormal liver tests to a more serious condition in which the fat in the liver leads to inflammation, scarring and cirrhosis, which is irreversible liver damage. NAFLD is very common and may be found in up to 1 in 5 adults. Of those with NAFLD, about 1 in 4 will develop the more serious form leading to cirrhosis. This is a very slow process and may progress over years to liver failure. It is related to obesity and as in the metabolic syndrome (see previous question) insulin resistance is the underlying cause. There is no proven treatment for this condition, apart from weight reduction, which results in rapid improvement in the abnormal liver tests. However in trials glitazones (see page 54) have been shown to improve liver tests and are beginning to be used in ordinary practice. Unfortunately they do have the effect of making people put on weight, which is often disappointing.

I was surprised when my doctor told me I had Type 2 diabetes as I thought this only occurred in people who were overweight and I am quite a slim person. My doctor says that because I do not need to lose weight, I will have to take tablets. Why is this?

It is true that many people with Type 2 diabetes are overweight but there are exceptions to this rule. People who are thin, especially if they have lost weight before diagnosis, are more likely to need tablets at diagnosis. They are also more likely to need insulin sooner rather than later.

Is diabetes a disease of modern times?

The earliest detailed description of diabetes was made more than 2000 years ago but it is much more common now than in the past. This is particularly true of Type 2 diabetes, which is becoming very common in some countries such as India. Diabetes in younger people is also becoming more common, and this has been related to increasing affluence and obesity.

My nephew, who is 11 years old, has just been found to have diabetes but has been started on tablets. I thought that all young people with diabetes had to take insulin injections.

Until recently, nearly all children with diabetes fell into the Type 1 group and therefore needed insulin treatment from the time of diagnosis. In the last few years, however, Type 2 diabetes has become increasingly common in children. This increase in Type 2 diabetes in the young is more advanced in the USA, where in some children's clinics more than half the children have Type 2 diabetes. This increase is related to changes in lifestyle of the population in general and young people in particular. To put it bluntly, the epidemic of obesity is the result of eating too much and taking very little exercise. Most experts feel that Europe is five to ten years behind America in the obesity epidemic (see Figures 1.3 and 1.4).

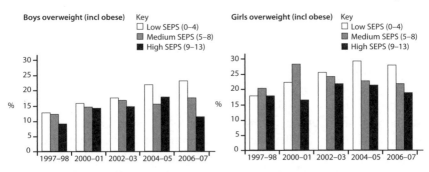

Figure 1.3 Prevalence trends in overweight and obese children (5–10 years) in England 1997–2007 according to social class. SEP score is a composite index taking into account income and social class.
Adapted from Stamatakis and colleagues, *International Journal of Obesity*. They show an encouraging fall in average weight in children (especially boys) from higher social classes, while disadvantaged children continue to have high risk of obesity, though the numbers are no longer rising.

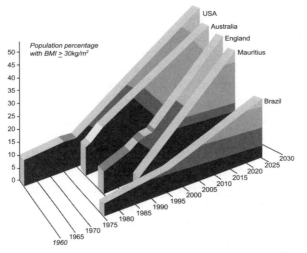

Figure 1.4 Projected prevalence of obesity in adults by 2025
Source: Adapted from National Obesity Observatory

Type 2 diabetes in children should be treated in the same way as in adults. First line treatment consists of an education package, which allows the child and parents to express their fears and helps them understand what this diagnosis means and what they can do about it. At some stages of the process, siblings should be involved as they will be affected by the diagnosis and may become useful partners in support of their brother or sister. The family should be encouraged to make changes in lifestyle and in particular decide how they can improve their patterns of eating. It is important to be shown how to monitor blood glucose in order to assess the response to any changes they make and to discover the effect of different foodstuffs and of exercise. Like most people with Type 2 diabetes, your nephew is faced with the prospect of taking increasing numbers of tablets to control his sugars and at some stage he will need insulin treatment.

Our 16-year-old daughter has just been found to have Type 2 diabetes. Apart from not needing insulin, are there any other differences between Type 1 and Type 2 diabetes?

It may come as a relief to be told that although your daughter has diabetes, she will not need insulin injections – at least for the time being. However, Type 2 diabetes is at least as serious a condition as Type 1. This is because young people with Type 2 diabetes, like adults with this condition, carry an extra threat of heart disease, though this will not apply to your daughter until she is much older. The risk factors include high cholesterol, triglycerides and blood pressure, and increased waist circumference (sometimes called the metabolic syndrome).

A study in America has looked at the frequency with which these risk factors appeared in different groups of young people aged 12–19 years. In the general population of American children, 6.4% in this age range had two or more of these risk factors. In young people with Type 1 diabetes, the frequency was 14%, while in those with Type 2 diabetes it was greater than 90%.

Although this information is bound to worry you, all these risk factors can be identified and corrected. It is important that your daughter has regular checks for body weight, cholesterol and blood pressure and if these are above the normal for her age, she should receive treatment to prevent or delay the risk of heart disease as she grows older. Some drugs used for treatment of cholesterol and blood pressure should not be used in pregnancy and your daughter needs to be aware of this.

My mother died very suddenly last year and not long afterwards I was diagnosed with diabetes. Can a bad shock bring on diabetes?

Sometimes diabetes develops soon after a major disturbance in life, such as a bereavement, a heart attack or a bad accident, and the diabetes is blamed on the upset. This is not really the case, as insulin failure in the pancreas takes a long time to develop. However, a bad shock can stress the system and bring on diabetes a bit earlier if your insulin supply is already running low.

I was very ill last year and developed diabetes, which has since got better. Can a severe illness cause diabetes?

Any serious medical condition (such as a heart attack or injuries from a traffic accident) can lead to diabetes. This is because the hormones produced in response to stress tend to oppose the effect of insulin and cause the glucose level in the blood to rise. Most people simply produce more insulin to keep the blood glucose stable. However, in some cases, if the reserves of insulin are low, the blood glucose level will climb. You had temporary diabetes, and the glucose level returned to normal once your stress was over. However, you will carry an increased risk of developing permanent diabetes later in life.

My latest baby was very big at birth. Would she have caused me to have developed diabetes?

No, the opposite is true. It is because you already had unrecognised diabetes that your daughter was big and any woman who has an unexpectedly big baby (more than 4 kg or 9 lb) should be tested for diabetes. If you had diabetes during pregnancy but your blood sugar returned to normal after your baby was born, you will continue to carry an increased risk of developing diabetes at some stage in the future. This is called gestational diabetes and you can read more about it in Chapter 7.

I have been found to have Type 2 diabetes. Is there anything I could have done to prevent this from happening to me?

Because of the epidemic of Type 2 diabetes in many parts of the world, a lot of work has been done to see if this condition can be prevented. Most people with Type 2 diabetes go through a phase of prediabetes, when they have slightly raised blood sugar levels without having full-blown diabetes. Large studies have been carried out in China, USA and Finland to see if training people to make life-style changes can prevent diabetes. In all three countries, the results were striking and showed that by restricting food intake and taking part in exercise programmes, diabetes could be held at bay. The recommended exercise was at least half an hour of fast walking or equivalent on five days a week. In the American study, some participants were asked to take a drug called metformin which increases insulin sensitivity and this also helped to delay the onset of diabetes. Metformin is widely used in the treatment of Type 2 diabetes (see question about metformin on p. 53).

A recent study which is still being analysed has shown that rosiglitazone, another drug which increases insulin sensitivity, reduces the chances of diabetes developing in people at risk. This was called the DREAM Study and involved 5269 people with 'prediabetes'. Those people who took rosiglitazone for the three years of the study reduced the risk of developing diabetes by 60% (see www.dtu.ox.ac.uk/dream/results for details).

My doctor said that the drugs I am taking for asthma might have caused my diabetes. Is this true?

Yes, several drugs in common use can either precipitate diabetes as an unwanted side effect or make existing diabetes worse. The most important group of such medicines are hormones.

Hormones are substances produced by special glands in the body and insulin from the pancreas is an example. Some hormones have been manufactured and found to be useful in the treatment of medical conditions such as severe asthma or rheumatoid arthritis. The most commonly used hormone drug is a steroid called prednisolone, which opposes insulin and therefore puts up the level of glucose in the blood. Steroids in large doses will often bring on diabetes, which usually goes away when the steroids are stopped.

The contraceptive pill is another steroid hormone with a mild anti-insulin effect. Sometimes people on insulin find that they have to give themselves more insulin while taking the pill.

Glucagon is a hormone from the pancreas with a strong anti-insulin effect. It is used to correct a severe insulin reaction (see the section *Hypos* in Chapter 3 for how and when to use glucagon).

Apart from hormones, some medicines, such as water tablets (diuretics) may have an anti-insulin effect and uncover diabetes.

I have recently been given steroid treatment (prednisolone) for severe arthritis. My joints are better but my doctor has now found sugar in my urine and tells me I have diabetes. Is this likely to be permanent?

Steroids are effective treatment for a number of conditions but they may cause side effects. One of these is to cause diabetes, which can sometimes be controlled with tablets (e.g. gliclazide). If large doses of steroids are being used, people often need insulin to keep the blood glucose under control. When you stop steroid therapy, there is a good chance that the diabetes will disappear.

However, you may have had diabetes without knowing it before you started on steroids, in which case you will still have diabetes after stopping steroids and will need to continue some form of treatment indefinitely.

I am told that other hormones that the body produces may cause diabetes. Is this true?

Diabetes occurs when there is not enough insulin for the body's needs. Sometimes excessive amounts of other hormones will tend to push up the blood sugar levels. If the body cannot respond with enough extra insulin, diabetes may result. Thus someone who produces too much thyroid hormone ('thyrotoxicosis' or 'hyper-thyroidism') may develop diabetes, which goes away when their thyroid is restored to normal. Thyrotoxicosis and diabetes tend to run together in families, and people with one of these conditions are more likely to develop the other.

Sometimes a person will produce excessive quantities of steroid hormones (Cushing's disease or Cushing's syndrome), and this may lead to diabetes (see the previous two questions for the connection between steroids and diabetes). Acromegaly is a condition where excess quantities of growth hormone are produced and this too may lead to diabetes.

I have had to go to hospital for repeated attacks of pancreatitis and now have diabetes. I am told that these two conditions are related – is this true?

Pancreatitis can be a very painful and unpleasant illness: it means that your pancreas has become inflamed. The pancreas is the gland that produces insulin as well as other hormones and diges-tive juices. If it is severely inflamed or damaged, it may not be able to produce enough insulin. Sometimes diabetes develops during or after an attack of pancreatitis and tablets or insulin are needed to keep control of the blood glucose. This form of diabetes is usually, but not always, permanent.

What other diseases would increase the chances of getting diabetes?

There are three groups of such diseases:

- Glandular disorders, in particular thyrotoxicosis (overactive thyroid), acromegaly (excess growth hormone) and Cushing's disease (excess steroid hormone, see above); polycystic ovary syndrome and fatty liver disease are both linked with insulin resistance and therefore carry an increased risk of Type 2 diabetes;

- Diseases of the pancreas, including pancreatitis, cancer of the pancreas, iron overload (haemochromatosis) and cystic fibrosis (a serious inherited childhood disorder); surgical removal of the pancreas (for either pancreatitis or cancer) also causes diabetes;

- Medical problems, such as heart attacks, pneumonia and major surgical operations which put stress on the body: the diabetes usually clears up when the stress is removed but these individuals may be more at risk of diabetes in the future.

You will find more information about the relationships between these disorders and diabetes in other questions earlier in this chapter.

Inheritance

My father had Type 2 diabetes. Am I likely to get it too?

Diabetes is a common disorder in this country and is diagnosed in about three in 100 people. A further two in every 100 have the condition without knowing about it – the 'missing million' – bringing the overall figure to about 5%. So in any large family more than one person may be affected, simply by chance. However, certain families do seem to carry a very strong tendency for diabetes. The best example of this is a whole tribe of native American people (the Pima): over half of its members develop diabetes by the time they reach middle age.

Genes are the parts of a human cell that decide which characteristics you inherit from your parents. The particular genes that you get from each parent are a matter of chance – in other words, whether you grow up with your father's big feet or your mother's blue eyes. Similarly it is a matter of chance whether you pass on the genes carrying the tendency for diabetes to one of your children. It is only the *tendency* to diabetes that you may pass on: the full-blown condition will not develop unless something else causes the insulin cells in the pancreas to fail. Unlike Type 1 diabetes, the actual genes that carry the risk of Type 2 diabetes have not been identified. Nevertheless, Type 2 diabetes has a much stronger family link than Type 1. If either of your parents has Type 2 diabetes, you have a 30% chance of developing prediabetes (see p. 13) and about 50% of people with this condition develop diabetes. So the overall risk is about 15%.

I come from an Indian family and number of my relatives have diabetes. I have been told that diabetes is more common in Asian families. Is this true?

It is an unfortunate fact that diabetes is much more common in families who originate from the Indian subcontinent. The risk seems to be related to moving from a subsistence life, where people have to work hard in order to grow enough food for survival, to a comparatively easy life of relative affluence, where food is easily available and hard physical work is no longer a fact of life. Indians who live in an urban environment have a risk of diabetes up to five times greater than that of a white person with a similar lifestyle. People of Indian origin who live in this country must be aware of their risk of diabetes, especially if parents and relatives are affected. As in all cases of diabetes, early diagnosis is vital if complications are going to be avoided.

I've been told that people from certain parts of the world are more at risk of diabetes. Could you tell me more about this?

C ertain groups of people have extremely high risk of diabetes. The Pima people, a native American tribe who live in Arizona, have a greater than 50% risk of diabetes. Other groups who have developed a sedentary lifestyle, such as South Pacific islanders from Nauru, who have grown rich, have almost as great a risk as the Pimas. Any population which exchanges a harsh rural environment for the relative affluence and inactivity of urban living carries a significant risk of diabetes. Thus rural Hispanics in the USA have a 7% risk of diabetes which increases to 17% in their urban counterparts. There is also a higher risk of diabetes in people of Afro-Caribbean origin.

Several members of my family developed diabetes when we were young and most of us are controlled by tablets. I've been told we are a MODY family. What does this mean?

M ODY stands for Maturity-Onset Diabetes of the Young. (Maturity-onset diabetes is an earlier name for Type 2 diabetes.) In the 1970s, it was noticed that a handful of families seemed to develop diabetes in their teens or twenties and about 50% of family members were affected. This suggests a certain sort of inheritance (autosomal dominant); those family members with diabetes have a specific defect in their insulin-producing cells. Research into these patients has increased our understanding of the causes of diabetes. There are several distinct types of MODY, but generally people in this group can control their diabetes with tablets and do not usually need insulin. Visit the website: www.projects.ex.ac.uk/diabetesgenes/mody/index.htm to find out more about this unusual form of diabetes.

If diabetes is known to be in my family, should I or my children take any preventive action?

T he inheritance of diabetes is a complicated subject and different types of diabetes are inherited in different ways. In Type 1 diabetes some family members may carry an increased risk, which can be identified by genetic testing. However, only a small proportion of the people who inherit this risk will go on to develop diabetes and no one has been able to pin down the factors that cause this to happen.

Type 2 diabetes is more strongly inherited than Type 1, and therefore often affects several members of the same family. It is now clear that a number of different genes are involved. The picture which is slowly emerging suggests that there are several different forms of Type 2 diabetes. The genetics of one rare form of inherited diabetes, called MODY, have been investigated in great detail and have increased our understanding of this condition but these discoveries do not apply to the vast majority of people with Type 2 diabetes (see MODY question above).

There is now evidence that family members who are at risk may put off developing diabetes by regular exercise, losing weight and sometimes by taking medication. They should have a blood glucose test as soon as they develop any relevant symptoms, so that diabetes can be detected and treated early.

I am 16 and have had diabetes for five years. Why has my identical twin brother not got diabetes?

A large 20-year research project has studied examples of identical twins with diabetes. The results show a difference between the way Type 1 and Type 2 diabetes are inherited. If you have an identical twin with Type 1 diabetes, you have only a 50% chance of developing diabetes yourself. On the other hand, if you had Type 2 diabetes (extremely unusual at the age of 11) your twin would be almost certain to get the same sort of diabetes. If your twin brother has not developed diabetes within the last five years, he has a very low risk of developing the condition.

SYMPTOMS

My partner was very thirsty before she was found to have diabetes. What was the cause of the thirst?

The most common signs of diabetes are thirst and loss of weight. These two symptoms are related and one leads to the other (there is more detail on weight loss in the answer to the next question). The first thing to go wrong is the increased amount of urine. Normally we pass about 1.5 litres (about 2 pints) of urine per day but people with uncontrolled diabetes may produce five times that amount. The continual loss of fluid dries out the body and the sensation of thirst is a warning that, unless they drink enough to replace the extra urine, they will soon become very dehydrated.

Of course people who do not have diabetes may also pass large amounts of urine. Most beer drinkers know the effects of five pints of bitter. In this case it is the volume of beer that causes the extra urine, whereas in diabetes the large volume of urine causes the thirst. In the early stages, the thirst is usually mild and most people fail to realise its significance unless they have had some personal experience of diabetes. Someone with undiagnosed diabetes will often take jugs of water up to bed, wake in the night to quench their thirst and pass urine, and still not realise that something is wrong. It would be helpful if more people knew that troublesome thirst may be due to diabetes.

I had lost quite a lot of weight before I was finally diagnosed with diabetes. Why was this?

The main fuel for the body is glucose, which is obtained from the digestion of sugary or starchy food. People with untreated diabetes cannot use this glucose as fuel in the normal way or store it. The unused glucose builds up in their bloodstream and overflows into the urine. Someone who has uncontrolled diabetes may lose as much as 500 g (just over 1 lb) of glucose (sugar) in their urine in 24 hours. Anyone trying to lose weight knows that sugar equals calories. These calories contained in the urine are lost to the body and are a drain on its resources. The 500 g of glucose lost are equivalent to 10 currant buns (2000 calories per day).

Lack of insulin means that the body cannot use glucose to provide energy or to build stores of starch and fat. As a result body tissues are broken down to form glucose and ketones (see the section *Urine* in Chapter 4), and this causes loss of fat and wasting of muscles.

My vagina has been really itchy and sore. My GP says it's to do with my diabetes. Can this be right?

A woman whose diabetes is out of control may be troubled by itching around the vagina. The technical name for this distressing symptom is pruritus vulvae. The equivalent complaint may be seen in men when the end of the penis becomes sore (balanitis). If the foreskin is also affected, it may become thickened (phimosis), which prevents the foreskin from being pulled back and makes it difficult to keep the penis clean.

These problems are the result of infection (commonly known as thrush) from certain yeasts, especially *Candida*, which thrive on the high concentration of glucose in this region. If you keep your urine free from glucose by good control of your diabetes, the itching and soreness will normally clear up. Anti-yeast cream from your doctor or pharmacist may speed up the improvement but this is only a holding measure while glucose is cleared from your urine.

I have had blurred vision for a few weeks and have just been found to have diabetes. Why has this affected my vision?

The lens of the eye is responsible for focusing the image on the retina. Blurred vision is usually a temporary change, which can be corrected by wearing glasses. The lens of the eye becomes swollen when diabetes is out of control and this leads to long-sightedness. As the diabetes comes under control the lens of the eye returns to normal. A pair of glasses fitted for a swollen lens at a time of uncontrolled diabetes will no longer be suitable when the diabetes is brought under control. If you have been newly diagnosed with diabetes and find that you have blurred vision, you should wait for a few weeks after the glucose levels have fallen before visiting an optician for new spectacles. The blurred vision may improve on its own and new glasses may not be needed.

Most of the serious eye problems caused by diabetes are due to damage to the retina (retinopathy). The retina is the 'photographic plate' at the back of the eye. Even minor changes in the retina take several years to develop but older people may have diabetes for years without being aware of it. In such cases the retina may already be damaged by the time diabetes is diagnosed.

In very rare cases the lens of the eye may be permanently damaged (cataract) when diabetes is badly out of control. This can be treated by removing the cataract and replacing it with an artificial lens.

See the section *Eyes* in Chapter 8.

Can diabetes be discovered by chance?

Yes, but this usually happens only in Type 2 diabetes. In Type 1 diabetes the diagnosis is more likely to be made because someone feels unwell and goes to the doctor.

In older people with no obvious medical problems, diabetes is often discovered as a result of a routine urine test – for example in the course of an insurance examination. Once the diagnosis is made, the person may realise that they have been feeling slightly thirsty or tired, but these symptoms may be so mild that they go unnoticed. However, even people who have had very few symptoms often feel they have more energy once diabetes is controlled.

Sometimes people are found to have diabetes when they suffer another medical condition such as a heart attack or a foot infection. In such cases diabetes, previously undiagnosed, has been the main cause of the new problem. The important message is that even though the symptoms may be minor, so-called 'mild' diabetes may lead to serious problems.

2 | Treatment without insulin

In this chapter and the next we describe different ways of treating diabetes. Most people diagnosed with Type 2 diabetes respond at first to changes in their diet. This alone may have a dramatic effect on their condition, especially in people who are overweight and manage to get their weight down. If changes in diet fail to control diabetes, tablets will be needed, but these will not work indefinitely and once they fail, insulin is the only alternative. A small number of people with Type 2 diabetes, who feel very unwell at the time of diagnosis, may need insulin immediately. Treatment with insulin is discussed in Chapter 3.

The most important thing for anyone with newly-diagnosed diabetes is to access good diabetes education. In the past, people were often given instructions about what to eat and which tablets to take without any explanation as to why it was important. Not surprisingly, they did not always follow the advice. The importance of structured education has been recognised in the national frameworks for diabetes (see p. 140), and education programmes have been developed for both Type 1 and Type 2 diabetes. The DAFNE programme was introduced for Type 1 diabetes in 2002, and following its success, a group of people interested in diabetes education started to develop a course for people with Type 2 diabetes. They devised the DESMOND programme – Diabetes Education Self Management Ongoing and Newly Diagnosed. DESMOND is available in 110 healthcare areas in UK and Ireland. While still designed for newly diagnosed patients with type 2 diabetes, the ongoing programme is now being put through trials (see www.desmond-project.org.uk). Eventually everyone with Type 2 diabetes should have access to a standardised education programme, which will help them to understand diabetes and make important decisions about lifestyle changes.

DIABETES EDUCATION

My doctor has just told me that I have diabetes and I am feeling very shocked and confused as I don't know much about it but I know it can be serious. My doctor has given me the telephone number of Diabetes UK so I can get more information but I would really like to talk to someone with diabetes. Can you help me?

Most people who are told they have diabetes feel very upset at the news. One of the problems is the uncertainty about exactly how diabetes will impinge on their life. We agree that a phone call to Diabetes UK helpline is a good idea; it has gone to a lot of trouble to produce useful information for people with newly diagnosed diabetes. However, the most important thing they can do is put you in touch with the local branch of Diabetes UK. Naturally these vary in their level of activity, but in some areas the local branch is very well organised to provide support and information to new members. This will give you the opportunity to speak to other people who are in the same boat.

Some GP practices have set up programmes for people with newly diagnosed diabetes and practice nurses are committed to providing high quality support.

What would really help you is group education, which has the added advantage of giving people the opportunity to share their experiences and provide mutual support. More areas are providing group education sessions and we hope that in the next few years structured education will be available to everyone with Type 2 diabetes.

I have had Type 2 diabetes for nearly two years and still feel rather uncertain about what this condition entails. A workmate has just been diagnosed and went to something called DESMOND. He was very impressed with the course and learned more about his diabetes in one day than I have in two years. Why was I not told about this?

As we heard in the previous question, people who have been told they have Type 2 diabetes are often left in the lurch with very little information and understanding of what difference it will make in their lives. The newly diagnosed part of DESMOND is now well-established and being taken up by more areas. The Ongoing DESMOND programme is being trialled in a number of centres and should become widely available in the near future. DESMOND is also being developed for use in other languages for people who do not speak English. The programme is based on recognised principles of adult learning. People are invited in groups of eight, with their partners if they wish. The sessions are run by two nurses or dietitians, who have been specifically trained to deliver patient education. Ideally people should have access to a DESMOND session within four weeks of diagnosis. Afterwards they should be able to identify their own health risks and set their own specific goals.

So far only sessions for the newly diagnosed have been fully developed (see Table 2.1) and a research project to test its effectiveness will soon be completed. The ongoing part of the programme, which is designed to provide continuing education, is being planned and will follow the same principles.

Other educational programmes have been developed, for example X-PERT. You should enquire whether structured education is available in your area and if so, should try to take part.

I have heard about the DESMOND programme and would like to take part in it. However I've been told that it is not available in my area. Is there any way I can get onto a course?

It is frustrating for everyone that it has taken so long to roll out DESMOND throughout the country. Fifteen centres in the UK took part in the pilot study for the DESMOND project early in 2004 and a formal research project was completed and published in 2008. However, it takes time to train the educators and put the structures in place to deliver the programme. Most difficult of all has been the problem of finding new money to fund DESMOND at a time when the NHS is in financial hardship. We know of one area where the local branch of Diabetes UK has joined with Lions International to raise money to pay for DESMOND courses. At the time of writing, 110 centres in the UK are signed up for DESMOND and the plan is that the course will be available to everyone with Type 2 diabetes. Some areas have adopted different educational programmes (such as X-PERT) and provided these have been properly evaluated, they will be equally valuable. Diabetes UK has recommended ways of assessing education courses and you can access this information from their website.

DIET

Knowing about the right type of food and the amount that you can eat is important. Most of the questions we have included help explain the general principles but people's diets are very individual, so do ask for help and further explanations from your own diabetes adviser or dietitian. It is particularly important to have an opportunity to review regularly what you are doing about diet. If you are looking for new ideas for meals, there are now many helpful recipe books written especially for people with diabetes, most of which are available from Diabetes UK. A list of current titles can be found in Appendix 1.

Table 2.1 DESMOND: topics covered at the newly-diagnosed patients' session with the time (in minutes) spent on each subject

DESMOND: newly-diagnosed curriculum	mins
Housekeeping	5
The patient story	10
What diabetes is	5
Main ways to manage diabetes	10
Diabetes consequences/personal risk	15
Monitoring and taking action	10
Food choices	20
Physical activity	5
Stress and emotion	5
Screening and annual clinics	5

There must be many people like me who have diabetes but who are not on insulin. Why have I been told to control my weight?

Achieving and maintaining a sensible weight helps the control of diabetes and also reduces other health risks such as high blood pressure and heart disease.

Over 80% of people who develop Type 2 diabetes are overweight. If you are overweight the insulin produced by your pancreas may be less effective. This is known as 'insulin resistance'. If you can reduce your body fat, your own insulin will become more effective and will lower your blood sugar. Insulin resistance is not only related to body weight but also to body shape. Your waist size indicates where fat is distributed and if your waist measurement is high (central obesity), insulin resistance and other health problems are more likely (see Table 2.2).

I'm sure I don't eat too much. Why do I keep putting on weight?

Our bodies need energy from food and drink in order to function. Extra energy is required for any additional activity e.g. walking, housework, climbing stairs, gardening. This energy is measured in calories or joules (see below).

To maintain a stable weight our energy intake (from food and drink) has to equal our energy output (for our daily activities.)

If your weight is increasing, your energy intake is exceeding your energy output, and the extra energy is stored as body fat. Even small differences in this balance will, in time, make a difference. An extra 100 calories (e.g. two small plain biscuits or one chocolate digestive) a day will amount to over 4.5 kg (over 10 lbs) weight gain in a year. Keeping a record of your food and drink intake can help you identify where you can make gradual changes, as your aim would be to reduce your food intake or increase your activity level, or ideally both.

In the UK we normally refer to calories, but some countries refer to joules: 1 calorie is equal to 4.2 joules. Strictly speaking, the proper term is kilocalories (often abbreviated to kCal) and kilojoules (abbreviated to kjoules or kJ). These are the units on the nutritional information labels on food packaging. Most people use the familiar term 'calorie' when they mean kilocalories, so this is what we have chosen to use in this book.

I have diabetes controlled by diet alone. Do I have to keep to strict mealtimes?

The vast majority of people on diet alone do not need to keep to strict mealtimes. However, you may find it easier to control your blood glucose and your appetite by spacing your food out into three smaller meals per day rather than having one or two larger meals. As long as you are on diet alone, your risk of low blood glucose (a 'hypo', see Chapter 3) is extremely rare.

Table 2.2 Definition of central obesity

Population group	Waist measurement
Caucasian (white) male	102 cm (40 inches)
Caucasian female	88 cm (35 inches)
Asian male*	88 cm (35 inches)
Asian female*	80 cm (32 inches)

*Asian people have higher risk than Caucasians so the waist measurement is lower.

My husband's diabetes is controlled by diet alone. Since being diagnosed two years ago, he has kept strictly to his food plan. In the past year he has not had a positive urine test and his blood glucose measurements at the clinic have been normal. Does this mean he no longer has diabetes?

Once you have developed diabetes, you have diabetes for life. Exceptions to this are extremely rare. Your husband has obviously done very well by keeping to his food plan, and at present this is controlling his diabetes. If he relaxed his eating plan, it is likely that his blood glucose would rise again and his diabetes would not be so well controlled. Diabetes is a progressive condition so in time your husband may require medication in addition to his diet but he should still be encouraged to maintain the improvements he has made to his food plan.

Do people whose diabetes is controlled by diet alone need to eat snacks in between meals?

The majority of people on diet alone do not need snacks in between meals. Having regular meals should be sufficient for most. If you are trying to keep your weight under control then having snacks may hinder your progress. However, if you are underweight and don't get enough energy from your meals then snacks may be useful.

There seem to be many foods offered in the supermarkets now labelled 'diabetic foods'. Should I be eating these rather than the ordinary types?

'Diabetic foods' do not offer any health benefits. They are expensive and are often no lower in fats or calories than ordinary food. They can still affect your blood glucose and can cause bowel upset.

In place of ordinary sugar these foods are sweetened with a substitute, often fructose or sorbitol both of which provide calories and can have a laxative effect.

Today the recommended food plan for people with diabetes includes some sweetened foods, especially if you choose products with a higher fibre and lower fat content. Depending on your glucose control and your weight, you should be able to eat small amounts of ordinary sweet foods, such as biscuits, cakes or sweets. These should form part of your food plan and should preferably be eaten at the end of a meal. There is no need for you to buy so-called diabetic foods to give yourself a treat.

The only 'special' foods we recommend for people with diabetes are the ones labelled as 'diet' or 'low calorie', e.g. sugar-free soft drinks, reduced sugar preserves, diet yoghurts and sugar-free jellies. These are not marketed specifically at people with diabetes, but for anyone who wants to keep their weight under control or avoid eating too much sugar. They are usually sweetened with intense sweeteners such as saccharin or aspartame which are virtually calorie-free. These artificial sweeteners can also be used to replace sugar in your tea or coffee, and are also available in granular form to sprinkle on breakfast cereal, or for use in baking.

Table 2.3 General nutritional information on food labels

	Per 100g	Per serving 200g	What this means
	TYPICAL VALUES		
Energy	232kJ 55kCal	464kJ 110kCal	Energy or calories from this food. Limiting total calories will help you lose weight
Protein	4.5g	9g	For body growth and repair. Most adults get more than they need
Carbohydrate *of which sugars*	8.9g 7.8g	17.8g 15.6g	Total carbohydrate includes both starch and sugar. Both will affect blood glucose. Sugars include natural (fruit and milk) sugars and added sugar
Fat *of which saturates*	0.1g 0.1g	0.2g 0.2g	Three main types: monounsaturates, polyunsaturates, saturates; all contribute high energy. Aim to eat fewer fats – especially saturates
Fibre	0.1g	0.2g	Important for good bowel function
Sodium	0.1g	1.2g	High levels associated with high blood pressure

Where or how do I find out about the carbohydrate or calorie content of foods?

There are many publications giving this information which are available in newsagents and bookshops. If you have access to the internet then a search will give you a great number of options. If you do not have access to the internet, your local library or Diabetes UKCareline may be able to help.

Another source of information is the nutritional labels on the foods you buy. If you find food labels difficult to understand then your

Table 2.4 Guideline Daily Amounts

Each day	Women	Men
Calories	Up to 2000	Up to 2500
Fat	Up to 70 g	Up to 95 g
Sugars	Up to 50 g	Up to 70 g
Salt	No more than 6 g	No more than 6 g

dietitian will be able to explain how to use this information. Tables 2.4 and 2.5 give some examples of what you may see on labels.

The guidelines (Table 2.4) are based on what an average person may have when eating a balanced diet. They are not therefore suitable targets for everyone. Individual requirements vary according to weight and activity level.

People often ask for figures of how much to look for on a label and Table 2.5 can provide some *guidelines*. It must be noted that the figures are per 100g of a food and each food choice should be taken in context of how much of it you eat and how often you eat it. No food needs to be excluded from an eating plan, but you should try and make sensible choices.

Many supermarkets have introduced labelling in traffic light colours (red, amber, green) to provide consumers with guidance on how healthy the food might be – green being the most healthy option.

I have just started tablets for my diabetes. Does this mean I can relax my diet?

You have been started on tablets for your diabetes because diet alone has not been enough to keep your blood glucose at a desirable level. Tablets are not a substitute for your diet but are an additional help, so it is very important that you maintain your efforts with your diet and with exercise. If you relax your diet then your blood glucose will be more difficult to control and your medication

Table 2.5 Further guidance on food labels

This is *HIGH*	This is *LOW*
Per 100 g	**Per 100 g**
20 g fat or more	3 g fat or less
5 g saturated fat or more	1 g saturated fat or less
0.5 g sodium or more (multiply by 2.5 = salt)	0.1 g sodium (multiply by 2.5 = salt)
10 g sugar or more	2 g sugar or less

may have to be increased prematurely in order to counteract your relaxed diet. This may also lead to weight gain. If it has been a while since you have seen a dietitian, it may help to make an appointment to review your food plan, now that you are on tablets, to discuss any other changes that you could make.

How does a person with diabetes get an appointment with a dietitian? Will there be one at my doctor's?

As diet plays a crucial part in the management of diabetes, it is important that you get sound expert dietary advice from a State Registered Dietitian. This is part of the recommended standard of care as detailed in the Diabetes UK booklet *What diabetes care to expect* (see Appendix 1).

The availability of dietitians varies across the country but most diabetes centres have a dietitian as part of their diabetes team. If you attend a hospital diabetes centre then you should be able to make an appointment with the dietitian. There are an increasing number of GP practices running local diabetes clinics and they should be able to arrange an appointment with a dietitian as part of your diabetes care.

I have a number of queries about my diet. Can you tell me how I can get advice about it?

If you have access to the internet you might try the Diabetes UK website which provides a huge amount of information which may help answer your dietary queries (www.diabetes.org.uk). It also provides a telephone service called Diabetes Careline UK: 0845 120 2960.

Good advice on diet is essential in the proper care of diabetes and it should be tailored to individual requirements. You may therefore prefer to arrange to see a State Registered Dietitian through your hospital or your GP. Most hospitals have a State Registered Dietitian attached to the diabetes clinic, and you could arrange to see them at your next clinic visit. Some general practitioners organise their own diabetes clinics, and may arrange for a dietitian to visit this clinic. Many nurses and health visitors who are specially trained in diabetes will also be able to provide good basic dietary advice.

I am a Hindu and have been diagnosed with Type 2 diabetes. Are there any specific dietary restrictions?

No, there are no specific dietary restrictions, except for keeping the amount of carbohydrates in your diet under control. You may need to eat smaller portions of rice, or fewer chapattis or rotis with your main meal, but there needs to be no change to the amount of meat or vegetables in your diet.

Avoid sweet preparations, especially gullab jamun, jillabee and similar sweets which have a very high sugar content, as these may cause your blood sugar to rise very quickly. Do not yield to temptation during religious festivals or at weddings when you will be offered a wide variety of sweets. Exercise regularly and keep your weight under control, as advised by your GP or practice nurse.

I am a Jew and I have Type 2 diabetes. Can you advise me on how best to cope with eating on the Sabbath?

Eating on the Sabbath (Shabbot) and holidays should be a happy time for families to gather together and celebrate. You will need to pay particular attention to the carbohydrate content of your meals and avoid food that is likely to increase your blood sugar level.

Jewish Law (Torah) restricts the testing of blood sugars on the Sabbath and festival days. So it is best to test either before or after the main meal the day before. This activity will be best carried out at a time when there are no guests around.

The Jewish Diabetic Association has a very active website which contains a number of articles and useful links on the glycaemic index of foods, recipes and healthy eating in the section on enlightened kosher cooking (www.jewishdiabetes.org). We strongly recommend David Mendosa's website: www.mendosa.com which contains helpful information presented in an upbeat style.

We are planning several family celebrations this summer and I would like advice on the choice of alcoholic drinks. I have managed to lose weight and my control has improved so much that I have been taken off my tablets.

Alcohol taken in moderation has been shown to have a positive effect on health. However, it does contain a significant number of calories, which can be a problem if you are trying to lose weight.

Your choice of alcohol is mainly a question of taste. More important than your choice of drinks is the quantity. Sensible recommendations are 3 units per day for women and 4 units per day for men. (For guidance on units see the section *Alcohol* in Chapter 5.) Exceeding this amount on special occasions will not have bad long-term effects. But a maximum weekly total of 21 units for women and 28 units for week for men is a sensible recommendation. We recommend sugar-free mixers as they will not increase your blood glucose and provide virtually no calories. Drinking alcohol affects your blood glucose level and you should be aware of this. It also contains a significant number of calories as shown in Table 2.6. There is more information about this in the section on *Alcohol* in Chapter 5.

Table 2.6 gives some guidelines, but remember that figures will vary with different brands.

Table 2.6 Alcoholic drinks

Drink	Serving size	Units of alcohol	Calories kCal	Carbohydrate or sugar
Spirits, e.g. whisky, vodka, rum, gin	25 mL	1	52	trace
Spirits, e.g. whisky, vodka, rum, gin	35 mL	1.5	73	trace
Lager, 3.5–4.5% vol (e.g. Tennent's, Fosters)	pint	2.2	166	10 g
Lager, premium, Special Brew	pint	4.5	338	14 g
Lager, alcohol free, bottled	300 mL	Trace	21	4.5 g
Beer (bitter)	pint	2.2	184	13 g
Stout, Guinness	pint	2.4	172	8.5 g
Cider, dry	pint	2.7	206	15 g
Cider, sweet	pint	2.7	240	25 g
Wine, dry white or red, 12.5% vol	125 mL	1.6	112–120	trace
Wine, dry white or red, 12.5% vol	175 mL	2.2	157–168	trace
Wine, med. white, 12.5% vol	125 mL	1.6	120	4.3 g
Wine, sparkling, 10% vol	125 mL	1.2	93	6 g
Sherry, dry, 20% vol	50 mL	1	58	trace
Sherry, med. 20 % vol	50 mL	1	58	3 g
Port	50 mL	1	79	6 g

I have had diabetes for 22 years and have only recently come back under the care of my local hospital. When I talked about my diet to the dietitian she was keen to make some changes, saying that there were quite a lot of new ideas and diet recommendations. Is it worth me changing after all this time?

Dietary advice has certainly changed a lot since you were diagnosed 22 years ago. As we learn more about food and how our bodies use it the advice about diet has to be adjusted. It is certainly worth knowing the new recommendations and it is never too late to make changes.

Dietary advice is now based on the principle of healthy eating which is encouraged for the population as a whole – not just for people with diabetes. The idea is that the whole family can be involved in good health rather than people with diabetes feeling they need a special diet. The major differences are an emphasis on:

- reducing fats, especially saturated fats;

- increasing fruit and vegetables.

There is now greater flexibility in choice: it is no longer forbidden to have sugar or sugary foods but advice is given on how much is recommended. We encourage carbohydrate foods which have a low glycaemic index (GI) (see glycaemic index question on p. 93) and recommend a reduction of salt and salty foods.

So it is worth updating your diet. Your dietitian will provide individual advice, suited to your lifestyle. The main recommendations are summarised in Figure 2.1.

I am gradually losing my liking for sweet foods. When I do have them I follow my dietitian's advice and make sure that it is at a time when they are least likely to result in high blood glucose. However, I really do not enjoy my selection of high-fibre breakfast cereals without some sweetener – I was a Sugar Puff fan before! Can I put a little sugar on?

It is quite all right for you to use a small amount of sugar on your breakfast cereal if you wish. The current dietary recommendations for diabetes recognises that up to 10% of your daily energy intake may be taken as sucrose provided that it is in the context of a healthy diet. However, if you would prefer to 'save' sugar for some other food, or to 'save' calories, then using an artificial sweetener would be the best alternative.

Figure 2.1

GUIDELINES FOR HEALTHY EATING FOR DIABETES

- Have regular meals – which include starchy carbohydrate foods such as bread, potatoes, rice, pasta, chapattis, cereals. We encourage high fibre starchy foods and foods with a lower glycaemic index (see Table 3.3).

- Cut down on fats – especially saturated (animal) and hydrogenated fats – trans fatty acids (found in some margarines, manufactured cakes and biscuits), both linked to heart disease. Use less butter, margarine, cheese, cream and fatty meats. Grill, bake or steam rather than fry. Trim fat from meat, skin from chicken and skim fat from stews and stock. Include oily fish e.g. salmon, sardines, mackerel containing Omega 3 fat which may benefit health. Choose lower fat dairy products e.g. low fat milk, low fat or diet yoghurt. If using oil, choose monounsaturated e.g. olive or rapeseed oil. Remember to limit hidden sources of fat such as pies, pastries, cakes and biscuits.

- Fruit and vegetables – aim for at least five portions each day – e.g. 3 vegetables and 2 fruits. These provide vitamins and fibre, are low in fat and calories. A typical portion would be 3 tablespoons of vegetables, 1 apple, 1 orange, 1 pear, 2 kiwis, 2 satsumas, 2 plums, small handful of grapes, 1 small banana. Avoid grapefruit or grapefruit juice if you take simvastatin to reduce your cholesterol.

- Reduce sugar and sugary foods. This does not mean avoiding sugar. A small amount of sugar in foods or in baking as part of a healthy food plan is acceptable. Choosing sugar free and low sugar drinks is recommended.

- Reduce added salt. A high salt intake can increase blood pressure, so avoid added extra at the table, reduce amount in cooking and limit high salt foods like cheese, bacon, salted snacks. Herbs and spices are a good alternative flavouring. A gradual reduction in salt is often the most acceptable approach.

Figure 2.1 (*continued*)

- Limit your intake of alcohol. The recommended intake is 3 units of alcohol for women and 4 units for men (see Table 2.6 for units of alcohol). Alcohol is a source of calories. Try to choose sugar free mixers. Alcohol increases your risk of low blood glucose, so it is sensible never to drink on an empty stomach.
- Aim for weight control. If you are overweight, losing weight will help with the control of diabetes and reduce other risks such as heart disease and high blood pressure. Reducing weight gradually and increasing activity is encouraged. Even a small amount of weight loss is beneficial. Waist size is an important indicator for health risk (see Table 2.2).
- We do not recommend diabetic foods such as 'diabetic' biscuits and sweets as they have no health benefits. They are expensive, can affect your blood glucose, are a source of calories and can cause an unpleasant laxative effect.

There are many artificial sweeteners on the market, both in tablet and granular forms. It's just a matter of taste what you choose. The tablet form of the intense sweeteners is calorie and carbohydrate free. The granular forms have a small amount of carbohydrate but because the product is so light and the portion serving is so small this will not have any significant effect on your blood glucose. Many supermarkets have their own brand names but some examples are Canderel, Sweetex, Shapers, Splenda and Hermesetas.

As a single parent I really find it hard to make ends meet. I know that very often I do not buy the foods that I should to help control my diabetes. Is there any way I can eat healthily but cheaply?

The food plan advised for people with diabetes should not cost more than the foods most people are eating before diagnosis.

Having said that, when people have limited incomes, the amount available to spend on food makes it more difficult and challenging to have a healthy diet. The following tips may help, and you could also ask your dietitian for some more ideas.

Planning meals ahead and making a shopping list will help you not to buy on impulse. Avoid shopping when you are hungry as you are more likely to buy items not on your list. Supermarket own brands are often much cheaper. Bread is often sold for less near closing time. (Avoid buying bargains if you cannot store them.) Bread, pasta, rice, crackers and porridge are cheaper sources of energy than sugary foods and are much healthier. Frozen vegetables can be cheaper and easier to use, as long as you have a freezer.

Fruit may look expensive but not when you compare it to cakes, biscuits and sweets. If you can get to a market the fruit and vegetables there can be cheaper.

- **Breakfast** Try porridge, which is healthy, cheap and excellent for diabetes control. When it's too hot for porridge, try muesli: supermarket own brand or make your own from rolled oats, nuts and a little dried fruit, or supermarket own brand high fibre cereal.

- **Lunch** A sandwich lunch can be very healthy, especially if you can use higher fibre, granary or pitta bread. Tinned sardines, mackerel or pilchards are healthy, cheap choices for sandwich fillings. Tinned fish, scrambled egg or beans on toast can also be inexpensive. Homemade soups with added pulses (e.g. lentils) are filling and are a good source of protein and fibre.

- **Main meal** You do not need large helpings of meat at your main meal, and you can often extend it by adding tinned tomatoes or other tinned, frozen or fresh vegetables or adding pulses e.g. beans and lentils. Diet yoghurts make excellent desserts and are good value for money. Another quick and healthy homemade dessert is a sugar-free jelly (available from most supermarkets), made up with milk or yoghurt, with fresh or tinned fruit.

The dietitian says that my high blood glucose levels during the morning may be caused by the pure fruit juice that I drink at breakfast. It is unsweetened juice, so how can this happen?

All fruit contains natural sugar and unsweetened fruit juices are no different. 'Unsweetened' means that the manufacturers have not added any extra sugar to the product. Many fruit juices are made from concentrated juice so can contain more sugar than the corresponding whole fruit. Juices are easy to drink and so your portion of fruit juice may be larger than you realise. Eating whole fruit is more limiting in quantity and because of the fibre content may produce a smaller effect on your blood glucose, but this is also dependent on the type of fruit or juice. It is acceptable to include fruit juice as part of a healthy diet but limiting the amount to a small glass at a time would be sensible. You can also dilute your fruit juice with mineral water or diet lemonade. You may prefer to choose a fruit juice with a lower carbohydrate/sugar content e.g. tomato juice or 'light' cranberry (which uses artificial sweetener).

My diabetes is treated by diet alone and I have headaches and a light-headed feeling around mid-day if I have been busy in the morning. I am all right after eating something. Why is this?

The symptoms you describe are similar to the feelings people have when their blood glucose is low – hypoglycaemia (see *Hypos* in Chapter 3). It seems surprising but some people on diet alone can go hypo if they go without food. This is because they produce their own insulin, but too late, and sometimes they produce too much. Ideally you should try to arrange a blood glucose measurement at a time that you feel odd in order to prove that you are actually hypo. If so, you could avoid the problem by eating little and often, especially on days when you are busy.

Overweight

I have just been told that I have Type 2 diabetes. Is it true that
if I lose weight I will probably not need insulin injections?

The majority of people diagnosed with diabetes have Type 2 diabetes and do not require insulin injections initially. Diabetes is a progressive condition and therefore it is not possible to guarantee you will never need insulin.

If you are overweight at the time of diagnosis then the first line of treatment would be to encourage you to reduce your weight and increase your activity. We know that weight loss can reduce insulin resistance (see the section *Diet*). So this approach will give you the best possible chance of delaying and possibly avoiding insulin therapy. Body shape is also important so losing weight from your waist area is encouraged. Targeting your activity to this effect would be very helpful.

If you are of normal weight at diagnosis, we would still encourage you to make changes to your diet and activity levels but there may be less scope for you to make a lot of changes, and you may progress to medication (tablets) and then to insulin more quickly.

I am trying to lose weight. How much should I lose a week?

It is best to lose weight gradually. If you are overweight then weight loss is to be encouraged but it is also important to keep the weight off. As you get used to the changes in your eating habits your new routine should become more familiar to you and make it less likely for you to lapse back to your old habits.

A target of 0.5–1 kg (1–2 lb) per week is realistic and achievable for most people. Losing weight more rapidly can cause you to lose valuable muscle as well as fat. To lose 0.5 kg (1 lb) a week you have to reduce your calorie intake by 3500 calories per week (500 calories each day). Increasing your activity will also help to use up some of these calories. You may find that you lose more in one week and less in another, but this is quite normal as your body adjusts to your new plan. It is important not to give up at these times and continue to maintain your efforts. By keeping a food diary and looking carefully at your choices and portions of food you can make your own aims for change. Even a small amount of weight loss (5–10%) is known to improve control of diabetes, decrease blood pressure and improve blood fats (e.g. cholesterol).

Fad diets may offer a quick fix but they are often unhealthy and most people find they cannot sustain them. It is common for people who lose weight too quickly to regain their previous weight *and more* within a few years.

> *I have been dieting on and off since I had my last child 15 years ago. The diabetes that I developed in that pregnancy has now returned despite the fact that I don't take sugar in my drinks. What more can I do?*

Having diabetes during pregnancy is called gestational diabetes and for most women it is temporary and resolves soon after the pregnancy. However, having gestational diabetes does increase your chance of developing Type 2 diabetes in later life. The dietary changes you have maintained (i.e. not taking sugar in your drinks) will have been helpful, but as you have had a cycle of dieting on and off over the last 15 years, our recommendation would be to aim for a more permanent lifestyle plan which would include a healthy diet and regular activity (see Healthy eating guidelines, Figure 2.1).

> *Why are both my dietitian and diabetes specialist nurse so against my family buying me diabetic foods? I find my diet very hard to keep to and never lose weight anyway. So why can't I have diabetic foods as a treat?*

Your dietitian and diabetes specialist nurse are not recommending the use of diabetic foods because those foods do not offer any health benefits. They are expensive and may affect your blood glucose. They are often high in fats and calories so will not help you lose weight. Finally they can produce an unpleasant laxative effect.

Having to follow any 'diet' is never easy and many people get fed up and find it hard to avoid what they perceive as forbidden foods. There are no forbidden foods for people with diabetes but we do recommend sensible guidelines. Having an occasional treat is perfectly acceptable but it is important to recognise *how often* you have a treat and *how much* you have.

If you feel frustrated by not losing weight then a better goal for you may be weight maintenance. As we get older our weight normally increases so not gaining weight is still success.

I am very overweight and trying hard to lose about 20 kg (3 stone). I love ice-cream and most of the cheaper varieties in the supermarket contain non-milk fat. Will this be suitable for me?

You can choose to include a small bowl of ice-cream as part of your diet plan. Non-milk fat means that the manufacturers have used cheaper vegetable fats, which provide just as many calories as milk fat. Most ice-cream contains about 7–10% fat and around 80–120 calories per (2 oz/60g) scoop – more in Cornish ice-cream. You can buy reduced calorie ice-cream but it is more expensive and you would have to decide if the saving in calories justified the cost. Like many foods it is helpful to identify how often and how much you eat them and aim to reduce the quantities and frequency in your efforts to reduce weight.

I have heard that there is a new appetite suppressant on the market but is it suitable for people with diabetes?

It is important to know that both appetite suppressant drugs that we discussed in the last edition are now no longer available

- Rimonabant was licensed for use in the UK in 2006 and was effective in helping people lose weight. However it turned out to carry a significant risk of causing depression and was withdrawn from world markets by the manufacturers in 2008.

- Sibutramine (Reductil) had been on the market for many years but was not recommended in patients with heart disease or hypertension. In January 2010, the government agency responsible for licensing drugs announced that Sibutramine should no longer be used as the risks of heart attack and stroke outweighed the positive effects on weight loss.

Although not an appetite suppressant, a further drug suitable for use in diabetes is orlistat (Xenical®). This works in the stomach and small intestine where it stops some of the fat from food being digested. This loss of fat is a loss of calories and therefore can aid weight loss. It is important that a low fat diet is followed to reduce unpleasant side effects. If you try this method of weight reduction, it is recommended that you make use of the telephone helpline provided by the company. This comes with a package to help you make changes in your lifestyle. It is disappointing that two promising drugs for weight reduction have been withdrawn but the encouraging news is that the new group of GLP1 agonists are often very effective in helping people to lose weight. They can only be used when other treatments for diabetes have failed and the main drawback is that they have to be injected – twice a day for Byetta and once a day for Victoza (see p 61).

I have the greatest difficulty losing weight and a friend has suggested that I should try joining Weight Watchers. Will they accept people with diabetes?

Weight Watchers and other slimming clubs can be very helpful to people who are having trouble losing weight, and that includes people with diabetes. They may ask for a letter from your doctor to confirm approval. We frequently encourage people to join a slimming club, as they are often very successful in helping with weight loss where other efforts have failed. They can also support you after you have reached your target weight and need to maintain your weight loss. Any club which helps you with your motivation is to be encouraged.

EXERCISE

I've heard that exercise is good for people with diabetes – is this true? If so, I'm not the sporty type and have never found going to the gym has any appeal to me. What should I do?

E xercise is good for people with diabetes (and for everyone else as well), and indeed it is one of the few things that have been shown to reduce the risk of developing diabetes. Exercise does not have to involve sports, and you can usually find something to suit your lifestyle. The staff at your local fitness centre are specially trained to help you with this, and these centres are a good place to start. They will work out an exercise programme with you and show you how to improve your fitness.

If you don't want to visit a fitness centre, here are some other suggestions.

- Walk whenever you can and avoid using the car.
- Climb stairs rather than take the lift.
- Walk to and from work.
- Take your dog for more or longer walks.
- Consider buying a bicycle or exercise bike.
- Make a point of taking at least three half-hour walks a week at a fast pace.
- Take up swimming.

I have been told that it is important to take exercise now I have been found to have Type 2 diabetes. I'm not sure exactly what I need to do. Could you give me some specific advice?

T he exercise programmes that have been used in large research projects were designed to prevent diabetes in people with a high risk. However, there is no reason why the same programmes should not be useful in treating Type 2 diabetes. The recommended time spent in exercise is 150 minutes a week, which is 30 minutes a day with a couple of rest days.

The type of exercise can be anything that makes you short of breath, such as fast walking, swimming, cycling, visiting a gym, dancing, taking up a sport or using an exercise machine. Choose a form of exercise which you find pleasurable. You may enjoy the experience more if you exercise with a friend or partner.

Exercise can of course bring down your blood glucose, and if you are using insulin you may need to reduce the dose before you are physically active. If you take a sulphonylurea (such as gliclazide) you should be on the look-out for hypoglycaemia and possibly reduce the dose if this happens.

If I keep to a good diet, why do I need to exercise as well?

Regular exercise stimulates a series of events in the body that result in changes in body composition. It reduces the amount of fat and increases the amount of lean tissue: muscle, fibres and bone. This increases your metabolic rate and improves your fitness, which is the amount of exercise that you can do without getting tired or exhausted. This not only makes you feel better but also reduces blood pressure and the 'bad' cholesterol (low density, LDL) and increases the 'good' cholesterol (high density, HDL). (See the question below on cholesterol.) Increasing fitness also increases the body's sensitivity to insulin and lowers blood glucose levels. It may also increase the tendency to develop hypoglycaemia and you might be able to reduce your insulin dose as your fitness improves.

I have been for a cholesterol check-up, but I noted that the doctor also wanted to check for different types of cholesterol. What's the difference between all these measurements and what do they mean?

Cholesterol is a fat (lipid) and an important normal component of many body tissues including hormones. Its concentration in the blood, where it circulates attached to a protein (hence it is called a 'lipoprotein'), has been shown to be a valuable indicator of the risk of developing vascular disease. High levels of cholesterol are associated with an increased risk of heart attacks. There are two major components of cholesterol known as low density lipoprotein (LDL) and high density lipoprotein (HDL). LDL is known as the 'bad' cholesterol as it is the most important risk factor for heart disease. HDL on the other hand is the 'good' cholesterol, since high levels of HDL are associated with a low risk of heart disease. Thus a 'high cholesterol value' is ambiguous unless you know whether it is high because of increased LDL or HDL cholesterol. This is important as HDL values may be high in people with Type 1 diabetes (insulin raises the HDL level) and as such do not indicate an increased risk of heart disease. Thus before contemplating any treatment for 'high cholesterol', your doctor needs to know that it is the 'bad' cholesterol (LDL) that is to blame. It's a complicated story and we hope that this explanation helps. Visit: www.lipidsonline.org for more information.

I have Type 2 diabetes and take the highest doses of metformin and gliclazide but am not well controlled. My doctor tells me that I could avoid insulin if I made a determined effort to improve my fitness and lose some weight. Is this true?

Yes, you may be able to postpone the need for insulin by becoming more physically fit and losing weight, though this is a tall order. Exercise has been shown to improve metabolic control in people with poorly controlled Type 2 diabetes. If you are to succeed, you will need to take up some form of regular exercise. The choice is best left to you and you should aim to take part in exercise five days a week which puts up your pulse rate above 100 per minute for half an hour. You could adopt a fitness programme and continue this regularly. However, there are any number of different ways of increasing your activity level such as brisk walking, dancing, swimming or gardening. It is important to plan in some detail how you will exercise. Don't forget that when it comes to the crunch, there will be many reasons why you *won't* want to take exercise at a particular time. It is worth trying to predict what these barriers might be in advance and work out ways round them.

If you wish to lose weight as well, you will need to combine this exercise programme with a calorie-reduced diet, as exercise by itself is not a good way of losing weight. If you want to pursue this line, you could visit your local fitness centre where they will be able to help you design a suitable programme, encourage you and monitor your progress.

TABLETS

I understand that there are different sorts of diabetic tablets. Can you tell me what they are and what the difference is between them?

There are five different types of tablet that may be prescribed for people with diabetes. They work in different ways.

- **Sulphonylureas** which include gliclazide, glibenclamide, glipizide and glimepiride. These act by increasing the amount of natural insulin produced by the pancreas.

- **Biguanides** are only available as metformin (Glucophage®). It works by reducing the release of glucose from the liver and increasing the uptake of glucose into muscle.

- **Thiazolidinediones** which include rosiglitazone (Avandia®) and pioglitazone (Actos®). These target 'insulin resistance' and are used in people who have been unable to control their blood glucose levels with metformin or a sulphonylurea. Both are also available in combination with metformin as Avandamet® and Actoplus Met®.

- **Alpha glucosidase inhibitor** (acarbose or Glucobay®). This slows the digestion of carbohydrates in the intestine and suppresses the rise in blood glucose after meals.

- **Prandial** (mealtime) **glucose regulators** which include repaglinide (Prandin®) and nateglinide (Starlix®). These stimulate the release of insulin from the pancreas and are taken with meals. They can be used on their own or with metformin.

I am taking gliclazide but am getting dizziness. Could the tablets be causing this?

G liclazide could be causing your blood glucose level to be too low so your dizziness could be a mild hypo, particularly if you get this feeling when exercising or before meals. You can easily confirm this by checking your blood glucose at a time when you feel dizzy. If your blood glucose level is above 4 mmol/L something other than gliclazide must be causing the dizziness. There are of course other causes of dizziness, which have nothing to do with diabetes, and if your sugar levels are normal, you should speak to your doctor.

I drop off to sleep all the time and never feel refreshed. I take 160 mg of gliclazide twice a day as well as 500 mg metformin. Could I be taking too much?

T his is quite a large dose of gliclazide and your sleepiness could be due to low blood glucose. You should use a meter to check that it is not below 4 mmol/L. On the other hand, people with high blood glucose often feel drowsy and lacking in energy. So your complaint could be due either to a low or a high blood glucose level, and you can find out by doing a blood glucose test. Speak to your doctor if the results are not in the normal range (4–8 mmol/L).

Since taking Glucophage, I have had feelings of nausea and constant diarrhoea and have lost quite a lot of weight. Is this due to the Glucophage?

Nausea and diarrhoea are possible side effects of Glucophage® (metformin). The loss of weight could be due either to poor food intake because metformin has reduced your appetite, or to your diabetes being out of control. Either way you should stop metformin or at least reduce the dose and see if the nausea and diarrhoea disappear. When you stop metformin, you may need a different sort of tablet or perhaps insulin injections. Your doctor will advise you.

My doctor wants to start a drug called metformin. He tells me this will protect my heart. Is this the case?

Metformin was discovered in France in 1958, so it is a well tried drug. It has well known side effects of diarrhoea, wind and tummy pain, which affect up to a quarter of those who try this drug. However, most people can tolerate it if they start with a low dose and always take it with food. There is some evidence from the UKPDS (see question on p. 109) that metformin provides protection from heart disease. Because of the side effects, metformin used to be second line treatment for Type 2 diabetes. Now that it is thought to give additional benefit, it's usually the first drug used when diet alone is failing. Metformin has also been shown to prevent the development of diabetes in people with prediabetes (see question on p. 13). It is also used in the treatment of polycystic ovary syndrome, a condition which is thought to be caused by insulin resistance.

My elderly mother has been taking gliclazide to control her diabetes for five years. Recently her sugars have been high and her doctor has asked her to take metformin as well with good results. Are there concerns about the long-term safety of metformin?

Metformin is a very good drug and we are not surprised that your mother's diabetic control has been better since she started taking it in addition to gliclazide. Metformin frequently causes side effects, mainly affecting the stomach or digestion (diarrhoea, constipation, nausea, loss of appetite). These side effects may develop after metformin has been taken for several years. However, many people have taken metformin for decades and there are no worries about its long-term safety.

What is the cause of a continuous metallic burning taste in the mouth? I am 62 years of age with diabetes, controlled on tablets for the last four years.

You are probably taking metformin tablets as these sometimes do cause a curious taste in the mouth. If the taste is troublesome you should stop taking these tablets. Other tablets for diabetes do not cause this side effect. You should consult your doctor for advice.

I have diabetes controlled on tablets. My dose was halved, and my urine was still negative to glucose. Would it be all right to stop taking my tablets altogether to see what happens? Obviously I would restart the tablets if my urine showed glucose.

Your idea is probably a good one, but you should discuss this with your doctor. You should also check your blood glucose level as urine tests can sometimes be misleading. Provided that your blood glucose remains controlled (between 4 and 6 mmol/L before meals and no more than 8 mmol/L two hours after a meal) it would be worth finding out whether you can control your blood glucose without any tablets. If this is successful, diet becomes even more important for controlling your diabetes and you must avoid putting on weight. Some people think that if they come off tablets, they no longer have diabetes, but this is not so. There is always the chance that they will need tablets or even insulin at some stage in the future.

I gather that there is a tablet for the treatment of diabetes called 'rosiglitazone'. What's different about it?

Rosiglitazone (trade name Avandia®, or Avandamet® in combination with metformin, from GlaxoSmithKline) acts by reducing the body's resistance to insulin. It is recommended as an additional therapy in combination with either metformin or a sulphonylurea (e.g. gliclazide or glibenclamide) when metabolic control is not adequate. The glitazones are now accepted as an effective treatment for Type 2 diabetes, although there has been some concern that rosiglitazone may be linked with an increased risk of heart attacks. A government regulatory body announced in July 2010 that the risks of using Avandia (rosiglitazone) outweighed its benefits and that 'it no longer has a place on the UK market'. Although the evidence against Avandia is not clear cut, it is probably sensible to use instead the alternative drug, pioglitazone (Actos), which is not thought to carry the risk of heart attacks. However it is well recognised that the glitazones may lead to fluid retention and so they are not recommended for people with heart failure.

I am about to go onto a glitazone and would like to know how it works.

You probably have Type 2 diabetes (see Chapter 1), not adequately controlled by your present tablets. Rosiglitazone was introduced in 1999 and pioglitazone (trade name Actos®, or Actoplus Met® in combination with metformin, from Takeda) soon after. They rely on the fact that Type 2 diabetes is caused by failure to produce insulin *and* resistance to the insulin that is available. Glitazones work by making you more sensitive to insulin so that whatever you can produce goes further.

Troglitazone was the first of this group of drugs to reach the market but it caused serious liver problems in a few people and had to be withdrawn. Extensive tests have been done on the new glitazones and they appear to be completely safe. However, most doctors like to arrange liver function tests when they first start people on these drugs.

Glitazones may be used as initial treatment in people who cannot tolerate metformin, or added to metformin, particularly if they are overweight. They may also be used in combination with metformin and a sulphonylurea. Side effects include weight gain, mild anaemia and fluid retention, which may sometimes put a strain on the heart There has also been an unexplained increase in the risk of fractures due to osteoporosis.

Unlike other drugs used for diabetes, glitazones work slowly and may take up to three months to have their full effect, so be patient.

I've just been put on pioglitazone and my blood glucose readings are no better – should I stop taking it?

Pioglitazone, like rosiglitazone, can be effective in controlling Type 2 diabetes. However, it does not usually have a rapid effect and you should wait at least three months before concluding that it is not helping your blood sugars.

I'm on rosiglitazone and gliclazide and my doctor wants to put me on metformin as well. Is this OK?

This combination of tablets is known as triple oral therapy. It is known to be effective and is sanctioned by NICE, the official government watchdog. In July 2010, another government body warned doctors against prescribing rosiglitazone, so you should probably use the alternative pioglitazone, which is believed to be safer. It is available as a combination tablet with metformin called Competact.

The downside of using triple therapy is the increased risk of side effects. Gliclazide rarely causes problems, apart from the risk of hypoglycaemia. Glitazones may lead to weight increase and fluid retention. Metformin is notorious for causing gastric side effects, such as nausea, diarrhoea and wind. Provided you are not troubled by these unwanted effects, you have a 50% chance of delaying the need for insulin. We do not want to give the impression that insulin treatment is a last ditch option, since many people with Type 2 diabetes do very well when treated early with insulin. However, some people are determined to stay off insulin as long as possible, either for psychological reasons or because they risk losing their job (see question on p. 159).

My doctor says my diabetes is not as well controlled as it should be and he wants to try a new tablet, sitagliptin, which he says will not make me gain weight.

Sitagliptin (Januvia) is one of a class of new drugs called DPP4 inhibitors (or gliptins), which have been developed to prolong the action of a hormone called GLP-1 (see p61). This hormone is produced by the intestines when food is taken into the stomach and one of its effects is to stimulate the pancreas to produce more insulin. GLP-1 is normally destroyed very rapidly by an enzyme known as DPP4 and if the action of DPP4 is blocked (by a DPP4 inhibitor) the effect of GLP-1 is prolonged for many hours. This enhances the blood glucose lowering effect of GLP-1. Unlike most tablets used to treat diabetes, the DPP4 inhibitors (gliptins) do not cause weight gain. Gliptins can be used in combination with any other blood glucose lowering tablet.

I have just started taking Glucobay tablets for my diabetes. Could you explain how Glucobay works?

Glucobay®, the trade name for acarbose, acts by slowing down the digestion of starch and related foodstuffs. Acarbose slows the breakdown and absorption of many dietary carbohydrates, reducing the high peak of blood glucose which can occur after eating a meal containing carbohydrate. It was launched in the UK in 1993, having been used very extensively in other European countries. It is an addition to diet treatment and has been shown to be effective in many people with diabetes who do not require insulin treatment.

I take Glucobay tablets but always feel very full and bloated afterwards. Would it be better not to take them?

Acarbose (Glucobay®) may lead to side effects when you first start taking it. These side effects are related to its action in the body (see the previous question). Because Glucobay slows down the breakdown of carbohydrates, complex sugars may then reach the lower part of the gut where they can cause a bloating sensation giving rise to wind (flatulence) and occasional bouts of diarrhoea. There are two ways of reducing this problem.

- Start with a very small dose of one 50 mg tablet of Glucobay a day, taken with the first mouthful of your largest meal. Increase the dose slowly, in consultation with your doctor, until the optimum dose is reached. This may be up to 100 mg three times a day.

- Try and exclude sucrose from your diet. Sucrose is the ordinary sugar that we add knowingly to sweeten food. It is also added to many foodstuffs by the manufacturers.

My doctor has recently started me on Prandin, which I understand is a new type of tablet for diabetes. How does it differ from metformin, which I also take?

Prandin® is the trade name for repaglinide, which, like nateglinide (Starlix®), is a prandial glucose regulator. This means that it controls the high glucose levels that can occur when food is consumed. It is a blood glucose-lowering tablet that stimulates the quick release of insulin from your pancreas at mealtimes, and should be taken just before a meal. If a meal is missed, the repaglinide should not be taken (unlike metformin). These tablets are usually used in combination with metformin. They should not however be used together with any of the sulphonylureas because they have a similar action.

I take a lot of tablets and have been told that I will probably have to change to insulin soon. What is the maximum dose of tablets I can take before insulin is required?

The minimum and maximum doses of tablets that you can take each day are shown in Table 2.7. Many people continue to use the maximum dose of tablets for years with rather poor control of their diabetes (HbA$_{1c}$ over 7.5%). Although these people often feel fairly well in themselves, they are usually much better off when they change to insulin – they have more energy and can usually manage on a less strict diet. In addition, running high blood sugar levels for years carries an increased risk of heart disease and other diabetic complications, such as eye problems.

What should I do if I am ill while on tablets? Should I take more or perhaps fewer tablets?

During the illness, you may not feel like eating, but you must not stop your tablets as any illness usually causes the blood glucose to rise. If your blood glucose readings are above 15 mmol/L, you should seek medical advice.

My doctor has advised me to change from tablets to insulin. Would I be right in thinking that I could avoid doing this if I cut down my intake of carbohydrate?

If you are overweight, you might be able to avoid insulin by dieting strictly and losing weight. If, on the other hand, you are a normal weight or underweight, you should not consider cutting back on your carbohydrate intake. Under these circumstances, you should almost certainly go onto insulin and will probably feel much better for it. Nowadays, Byetta and Victoza may be alternatives to insulin. They need to be injected but encourage weight loss.

My diabetes has been treated with tablets for two years and now my doctor has said I need insulin injections. Is my diabetes getting worse?

If your blood glucose can no longer be controlled with tablets, then your pancreas is becoming even less efficient in producing insulin, and in that sense your diabetes is worse. However, it does not mean that you are going to suffer any new problems from the condition, nor does it necessarily mean that you have done anything wrong. Diabetes

Table 2.7 Diabetes tablets

Name	Trade name (*)	Dose range (mg) per day
Sulphonylureas *(taken once or twice daily)*		
glibenclamide	Daonil, Semi-Daonil, Euglucon, Diabetamide, Gliken	2.5–15
gliclazide	Diamicron, Diaglyk	40–320
glipizide	Glibenese, Minodiab	2.5–40
glimepiride	Amaryl	1–6
DPP4 inhibitors (gliptins)		
Sitagliptin, vildagliptin, saxagliptin		15–180
Biguanide *(taken 2–3 times daily)*		
metformin	Glucophage	500–3000
Alpha glucosidase inhibitor *(taken 3 times daily)*		
acarbose	Glucobay	50–600
Thiazolidenedione *(taken 1–2 times daily)*		
rosiglitazone*	Avandia	4–8
rosiglitazone*/metformin	Avandamet combination	4/1000–8/2000
pioglitazone	Actos	15–30
pioglitazone/metformin	Actoplus Met	15/500–15/850
Prandial glucose regulators *(taken up to 4 times daily)*		
repaglinide	Prandin	0.5–16
nateglinide	Starlix	60–360

* Rosiglitazone will probably be withdrawn in September 2010.

is a progressive condition and many people will eventually move onto insulin. Once you have got over the initial fear of injecting yourself (and most people manage this very quickly) going onto insulin should not alter your life – in fact it will probably make you feel much better.

My mother is quite elderly and may have to take insulin. Are there new ways of giving insulin that will make it simpler for her?

Insulin administration devices such as Innolet have made it easier for older people to administer insulin. However, it is often difficult to predict whether an older person will be better off on insulin rather than tablets. The factors that her doctor will take into consideration are as follows:

- How unwell or thirsty does she feel while on tablets?
- What side effects are the tablets causing?
- How high are her blood sugars?
- How active and dexterous is she?
- How keen is she to start insulin?

Of all these questions, the last one is the most important. Older people must not be pressurised into starting a form of treatment which they dread. One way round this is to try insulin for a specified period, for example two months, and allow her to decide after that time whether or not she wishes to continue with insulin or revert to her previous treatment with tablets.

INJECTIONS OTHER THAN INSULIN

My doctor tells me that there is a new treatment for diabetes, which has to be given by injection but can help me lose weight. I have always resisted insulin because I was afraid of gaining weight, and I wonder if this new treatment might be the solution.

The new treatment you are talking about has been developed from a hormone known as GLP-1 (glucagon-like peptide). This is one of a group of hormones produced in the gut, which have four actions:

- stimulation of insulin production in response to food
- inhibition of glucagon (a hormone which increases glucose production)
- slowing of the rate at which food passes through the stomach
- an effect on the brain which reduces the appetite.

The overall effect is to reduce calorie intake with resulting weight loss and to reduce the blood glucose – a combination with great potential in the treatment of type 2 diabetes. GLP-1 can be used alongside established treatments but it does need to be given by injection. There are two preparations of GLP-1:

- Exenatide – Byetta (produced by Lilly) was launched in the US in 2005 and was licensed in the UK in 2007. It needs to be taken twice a day but unfortunately some people find it causes nausea and vomiting.

- Liraglutide - Victoza (produced by Novo Nordisk) is a similar drug which was licensed in 2009 and only needs to be taken once a day. It has similar side effects.

My wife is taking Victoza and for the first week or so was very sick. She now feels better but only eats very small meals and I am worried that she will become undernourished, because she is losing weight rapidly. Should she continue with Victoza?

Victoza (and Byetta) both work in a similar fashion by increasing insulin from the pancreas and reducing glucagon (see previous question). They also slow the rate at which the stomach empties and have a direct effect on the brain to suppress the appetite. These last two effects cause people to feel full and consequently they eat smaller portions. As your wife continues to lose weight, her diabetes should come under better control and she may be able to reduce any other medication she is taking for diabetes. Many people who lose a lot of weight while taking Victoza feel more energetic and more positive about life. We would recommend that your wife continue with Victoza under medical supervision.

NON-MEDICAL TREATMENTS

Recently I saw a physical training expert demonstrating a technique for achieving complete relaxation. She concluded by saying 'Of course, this is not suitable for everyone, for example people with diabetes.' Is this true and, if so, why?

This sounds like an example of ignorant discrimination. There is no reason why people with diabetes should not practise complete relaxation if they want to. If the session went on for a long time, you might have to miss a snack or even a meal but as you are burning up so little energy in a relaxed state, it should not matter.

My back has troubled me for many years and a friend has suggested that as a last resort I should try acupuncture. Would there be any objection to this, given that I have diabetes? Might it even help my diabetes?

Acupuncture has been a standard form of medical treatment in China for 5000 years. In the last 20 years it has become more widely used in this country. In China acupuncture has always been thought of as a way of preventing disease and is considered less effective in treating illness. In the UK acupuncture tends to be used by people who have been ill (and usually in pain) for a long time. It is most often tried in such conditions as a painful back, where orthodox medicine has failed to help. Even practitioners of the art do not claim that acupuncture can cure diabetes, but it will not do it any harm either, provided that you do not alter your usual diabetes treatment while you are having your course of acupuncture. If you have neuropathy (see Chapter 8) and have little sensation, it may be sensible to avoid acupuncture in the affected areas.

Do you think that complementary or alternative medicine can help people with diabetes?

A lternative medicine suggests a form of treatment that is taken in the place of conventional medical treatment. As such this could potentially be very dangerous, particularly if your diabetes is treated with insulin.

However, there may be a place for complementary therapies that can be tried alongside conventional medicine. Although there is no scientific evidence to show that complementary therapies such as yoga, reflexology, hypnosis or aromatherapy can benefit someone with diabetes, some people who have tried them report that they feel more relaxed. As stress can have a detrimental effect on blood glucose control, it may mean that their diabetes improves as a result.

We must emphasise that these therapies should always be used in addition to, not instead of, your usual diabetes treatment. You should not alter your recommended diet or stop taking your tablets or your insulin, nor would a reputable complementary practitioner suggest that you do any of these things.

I have heard that there are herbal remedies for diabetes. What would these be?

T here are many plants that have been said to reduce the high level of blood glucose in people with diabetes. One of these is a berry from West Africa and another a tropical plant called karela or bitter gourd. The problem is that to get any significant effect you need to consume more karela than is realistic. Consequently, it has only a minimal effect on lowering blood glucose and, as the bitter gourd lives up to its name and tastes disgusting, you will find conventional tablets more convenient, more reliable and safer. Herbal remedies have no beneficial effect on diabetes treated with insulin.

> *I recently read an article on ginseng that said it was beneficial to people with diabetes. Have you any information on this?*

Ginseng comes from Korea and the powdered root is said to have amazing properties. There is no scientific evidence to suggest that it is of any help to people with diabetes.

> *An evangelistic healing crusade claims to heal among other diseases 'sugar diabetes', malignant growth and multiple sclerosis, etc. Are these claims correct?*

There are, of course, a handful of (unproven) reports of miracle cures of various serious diseases like cancer, but these are few and far between. A mildly overweight person might be persuaded to lose weight by a faith healer and so it might appear that the diabetes was 'cured', but no person on insulin has ever benefited from a healing crusade except in the strictly spiritual sense.

3 | Treatment with insulin

Insulin was discovered by Frederick Banting and Charles Best in the summer of 1921. The work was carried out in the Physiology Department of Toronto University while most of the staff were on holiday. Before insulin was discovered, there was no treatment for people with diabetes and if they had what we now call Type 1 diabetes, death was inevitable, usually within a year of diagnosis. The first human to be given insulin was a 14-year-old boy named Leonard Thompson who was dying of diabetes in Toronto General Hospital. This was an historic event, representing the beginning of modern treatment for diabetes. It was then up to the chemists to transform the production of insulin into an industrial process on a vast scale.

There are two groups of people who need insulin. The first group are severely insulin deficient and cannot survive without it (Type 1 diabetes, see p. 5). The other group tends to develop diabetes later in life and they continue to produce some insulin (Type 2 diabetes, see p. 6). These people can usually be treated with diet and tablets initially but need insulin sooner or later. Treatment without insulin is covered in Chapter 2.

Insulin still has to be given by injection because at present it is inactivated if taken by mouth. Inhaled insulin has just been released but it not available for general use in the UK (see question on inhaled insulin, p. 68). About a quarter of all people with diabetes are treated with insulin. Virtually everyone who develops diabetes when they are young needs insulin from the time of diagnosis. People diagnosed in later life may manage quite satisfactorily for many years on other forms of treatment but eventually many of them will need insulin to supplement the diminishing supply of insulin from their pancreas.

Most people dislike the thought of having to inject themselves but modern insulin pens and needles are so well designed that these fears usually disappear after the first few injections. In general, insulin injections become part of the daily routine.

TYPES OF INSULIN

Since the discovery of insulin, countless people with diabetes have injected themselves with insulin extracted from the pancreas of cows and pigs. In the last 20 years or so human insulin has become widely available. However, human insulin is not extracted from human pancreas in the same way beef or pork insulin is. A great deal of research went into producing 'human' insulin by means of genetic engineering. This means that the genetic material of a bacterium or a yeast is reprogrammed to make insulin instead of the proteins it would normally produce. The insulin manufactured in this way is rigorously purified and contains no trace of the original bacterium.

The first insulin to be made was clear soluble insulin also called short-acting insulin. Injected under the skin, this insulin works within about 30 minutes and lasts for 4–8 hours. Various modifications were made to this original insulin so that it would last longer after injection. When protamine or zinc is incorporated into the soluble insulin, a single injection could last from 12 to 36 hours. For many years a single daily injection was advised by doctors, but people realised that this was not a good way of controlling the variations in blood glucose that occur during the day. Nowadays many people who need insulin have a mixture of short- and intermediate- or long-acting insulin twice a day, but an increasing number have insulin four or more times a day, injected using an insulin pen (see the section *Insulin pens* later in this chapter). A new generation of insulins, also called insulin analogues, where the chemical make-up of the insulin is changed, are also available today. By changing the molecular structure of the insulin, manufacturers can alter the way it works, allowing it to be absorbed differently.

I have recently heard that human insulin can be dangerous, although I've taken it for several years. Should I be worried?

There has been adverse publicity about human insulin. A number of people changing from animal to human insulin have noticed that they get less warning of hypos. This change of awareness may result from other factors (see the section *Hypos* later in this chapter) but some people are convinced that the problem was caused by human insulin.

There have also been reports of unexpected deaths in people who have changed to human insulin. These deaths may have been due to a low blood glucose but this has not been proved. Nor has it been shown that the numbers involved have increased since human insulin was introduced. Diabetes UK has been carrying out research into these vital questions but so far no cause for alarm has been found.

I am a Muslim and have been put on insulin. I hear that this is made from pork. Is this right?

Yes and no. Some insulins are pork-based, and there are pork-based synthetic insulins, both of which are unacceptable to Muslims. You need to inform your doctor or nurse of your wishes, stating that you wish to use a non-porcine synthetic (human) insulin instead. 'Human insulin' is not manufactured from human tissue, but is so called because it is 'akin to human'.

> *I've had diabetes for ten years and still hate giving insulin injections. I hear that at last inhaled insulin is available. How do I get hold of it?*

Inhaled insulin (Exubera – Pfizer) became available in USA and UK in 2006 after a great deal of time and money was spent on developing it. There were serious restrictions on its use in this country. It did sound like the answer to many people's prayers especially those with needle phobia. However, there were problems with giving insulin into the lungs and difficulties in achieving accurate doses by this route. There was also a worry that inhaling large quantities of a protein on a regular basis may lead to lung damage or even cancer. In October 2007, the manufacturers decided to stop making and selling inhaled insulin because it failed to 'gain acceptance among patients and physicians'. Other companies who were developing their own forms of inhaled insulin dropped their interest in these projects.

Inhaled insulin is not recommended for the routine treatment of people with Type 1 or Type 2 diabetes mellitus.

Inhaled insulin may be used as a treatment option for people with Type 1 or Type 2 diabetes mellitus who show evidence of poor glycaemic control despite other therapeutic interventions (including, where appropriate, diet, oral hypoglycaemic agents [OHAs] and subcutaneous insulin) and adequate educational support, and who are unable to initiate or intensify pre-prandial subcutaneous insulin therapy because of either:

- a marked and persistent fear of injections that meet DSM-IV criteria for specific phobia 'blood injection injury type' diagnosed by a diabetes specialist or mental health professional;

- severe and persistent problems with injection sites (for example, as a consequence of lipohypertrophy) despite support with injection site rotation.

In patients receiving inhaled insulin under the circumstances set out above, treatment should only be continued beyond six months, and in the longer term, if there is evidence of a sustained improvement in glycated haemoglobin(HbA$_{1c}$) that is judged to be clinically relevant to the individual patient's overall risk of developing long-term complications of diabetes.

Initiation of inhaled insulin treatment and monitoring of response should be carried out only by a specialist centre.

(NICE 12 October 2006. Final Appraisal Determination Diabetes [Type 1 and 2], Inhaled Insulin)

There seem to be a lot of different types of insulin on the market. Can you give me some details?

The range of insulins available can be confusing, although they do fall into four separate groups which are shown in Table 3.1. The times of insulin action vary greatly from one person to another and those given must only be regarded as a rough guide.

The vials mentioned in the table are bottles of insulin for use with a syringe, and cartridges are for use with an insulin pen.

I am taking a mixture of short- and intermediate-acting insulin twice a day and do not understand which insulin is working at which time of day.

Many people are confused by the length of action of their insulin particularly when taken more than twice a day. The diagram in Figure 3.1 gives a representation of some commonly used regimens. However, as a general rule the short-acting insulin works rapidly (morning and evening) and the intermediate-acting insulin takes longer and covers the afternoon and the night. If you are still unclear about it have another word with your doctor or diabetes specialist nurse.

Table 3.1 Insulins available in the UK (August 2010)

Rapid-acting (analogue) insulin which is clear, has an onset of action within 15 minutes, a peak action of 30–70 minutes and lasts 2–5 hours

Name	Manufacturer	Source	Vial or cartridge*	Prefilled pen
Humalog	Lilly	Analogue	Cartridge and vial	Humalog Pen
NovoRapid	Novo Nordisk	Analogue	Cartridge	Flexpen
Apidra	Sanofi-Aventis	Analogue	Cartridge and vial	Optiset Pen

Soluble insulin which is clear, has an onset of action around 30 minutes, a peak action of 2–3 hours and lasts for 4–6 hours

Name	Manufacturer	Source	Vial or cartridge	Prefilled pen
Humulin S (Soluble)	Lilly	Human	Cartridge and vial	No
Insuman Rapid	Sanofi-Aventis	Human	Cartridge	Optiset Pen
Actrapid	Novo Nordisk	Human	Vial	No
Hypurin Porcine Neutral[†]	Wockhardt UK	Pork	Cartridge and vial	No
Hypurin Bovine Neutral[†]	Wockhardt UK	Beef	Cartridge and vial	No
Velosulin (until Dec. 2007)	Novo Nordisk	Human	Vial	No

* Vials are bottles of insulin for use with a syringe, and cartridges are for use with an insulin pen

Intermediate acting insulin which is cloudy and lasts 6–24 hours with a peak action of 4–8 hours

Name	Manufacturer	Source	Vial or cartridge	Prefilled pen
Humulin I (isophane)	Lilly	Human	Vial and cartridge	Humulin I Pen
Insulatard	Novo Nordisk	Human	Vial and cartridge	Innolet
Insuman Basal	Sanofi-Aventis	Human	Vial and cartridge	Optiset Pen
Porcine Insulatard (until Dec. 2007)	Novo Nordisk	Pork	Vial	No
Hypurin Porcine Isophane†	Wockhardt UK	Pork	Vial and cartridge	No
Hypurin Bovine Isophane†	Wockhardt UK	Beef	Vial and cartridge	No

Intermediate/ Long-acting analogue insulin which is clear and lasts between 12 and 24 hours with no peak action

Name	Manufacturer	Source	Vial or cartridge	Prefilled pen
Levemir	Novo Nordisk	Analogue	Cartridge	Flexpen
Lantus	Sanofi-Aventis	Analogue	Vial and cartridge	Optiset Pen

Long-acting insulin

Name	Manufacturer	Source	Vial or cartridge	Prefilled pen
Hypurin Bovine Lente†	Wockhardt UK	Beef	Vial	No
Hypurin Bovine PZI†	Wockhardt UK	Beef	Vial	No

Table 3.1 Insulins available in the UK (August 2006) *continued*

Mixed insulin containing short-acting and intermediate-acting insulin in varying proportions*

Name	Manufacturer	Source	Vial or cartridge	Prefilled pen
Mixtard 30 (to be withdrawn in 2010)	NovoNordisk	Human	Cartridge	Innolet
Mixtard 50 (until Dec. 2007)	NovoNordisk	Human	Cartridge	No
Humulin M3	Lilly	Human	Vial and cartridge	Humulin M3 Pen
Insuman Comb 15	Sanofi-Aventis	Human	No	Optiset Pen
Insuman Comb 25	Sanofi-Aventis	Human	Vial and cartridge	Optiset Pen
Insuman Comb 50	Sanofi-Aventis	Human	Cartridge	Optiset Pen
Porcine Mixtard 30 (until Dec. 2007)	NovoNordisk	Pork	Vial	No
Hypurin Porcine Mix 30/70†	Wockhardt UK	Pork	Vial and cartridge	No

Mixed insulin comprising rapid-acting analogue insulin and intermediate-acting analogue insulin

Name	Manufacturer	Source	Vial or cartridge	Prefilled pen
Humalog Mix 25**	Lilly	Analogue	Cartridge	Humalog Mix 25 Pen
Humalog Mix 50**	Lilly	Analogue	Cartridge	Humalog Mix 50 Pen
Novomix 30¶	Novo Nordisk	Analogue	Cartridge	Flexpen

† All Hypurin packaging is marked with braille

* The numbers refer to the percentage of soluble (short-acting) to isophane (intermediate-acting) insulin, e.g. Humulin M3 is 30% soluble to 70% isophane

** Humalog mixes are a mixture of lispro solution and lispro protamine suspension (both analogue insulins)

¶ NovoMix 30 is 30% soluble insulin aspart and 70% insulin aspart protamine

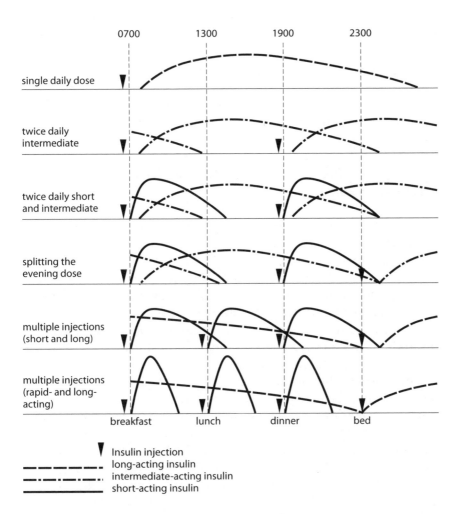

Figure 3.1 Five common insulin regimens

Can I get AIDS from human insulin?

Definitely not. Human insulin is made either from bacteria or yeast 'instructed' to produce insulin that has the same structure as human insulin, or from pork insulin modified to resemble human insulin. It is rigorously purified and cannot be a source of infection.

Is it possible to be allergic to insulin?

Very occasionally people may develop an allergy to one of the additives to insulin such as protamine or zinc, but the insulin itself is unlikely to cause an allergy.

My doctor wants me to change to four injections a day. Is this necessary?

More and more people are taking four injections a day and in general they are happy with this arrangement, even though it obviously means more injections. Twice-daily insulin is a compromise with each injection containing a mixture of short- and long-acting insulin in the hope that this will provide the correct amount of insulin for each meal and the times in between eating.

We all need a small amount of insulin to trickle into our body throughout the day to keep our glucose level steady. We sometimes call this background (or basal) insulin and for people who are of a normal weight, this usually amounts to up to 24 units a day. The amount of background insulin needed varies under different circumstances, such as exercise, illness and after drinking alcohol, to name but a few. On top of this background insulin, we also need insulin with every meal (bolus insulin) to deal with the effects of food on the blood sugar. The actual amount of insulin needed depends on the type of food and in particular the amount of carbohydrate eaten. Your dietitian or diabetes specialist nurse should be able to give you general advice on this topic.

Would I be able to achieve better control if I went onto three injections a day?

If you are on two insulin injections a day, you probably take a premixed insulin such as Mixtard before breakfast and before your evening meal. It is possible to achieve good control with this sort of insulin, but many people find that they are unable to keep their sugars down at a certain time of day without running the risk of hypos at another time. This is a built in problem with fixed mixtures of insulin. Most commonly, sugars are high at bedtime after a good evening meal. If this is the case, we suggest 'splitting the evening dose' of insulin by having short-acting insulin before your evening meal and long-acting insulin at bedtime. This will allow you to adjust the dose of each insulin to achieve good results without going hypo in the night.

I have heard people refer to 'basal bolus' insulin. What does this mean and is it effective?

Basal insulin is needed to maintain a normal blood sugar, when the body is in a basal or resting state. This varies depending on the time of day and may be affected by illness and other conditions. It is normally given in the form of a long-acting insulin at night, which should last for 24 hours. If it fails to achieve this, another dose of long-acting insulin can be given in the morning. The word bolus comes from the Latin, meaning a cast of the dice or a lump: this refers to the insulin given before you eat to control the effect of food you are about to take in. This is normally a short-acting insulin or very short-acting analogue. This combination is now widely used in Type 1 and Type 2 diabetes and gives people the greatest flexibility in what they eat and when they eat it.

TIMING

I have been taking a combination of tablets and insulin and my doctor now wants me to change to two or even four insulin injections a day. Will this interfere with my social life – eating out, and so on?

No, on the contrary, more injections should make your life more flexible. Most people on one injection a day find that they need a meal in the late afternoon, around 6–7 p.m. With a second injection, this meal can be delayed for several hours with the insulin given shortly beforehand. With an insulin pen, it is more convenient to give yourself an insulin injection when eating out.

I have heard that there is a new fast-acting insulin which is even faster-acting than Actrapid. Does it have any advantages?

You are quite right, there are now five new synthetic 'designer' insulins: three rapid-acting insulins – lispro (Humalog®), aspart (NovoRapid®) and Apidra® from Aventis. There are also two longer-acting versions: glargine (Lantus®) and detemir (Levemir®) They are the first of what will be a series of new insulins (known as insulin analogues) which will be produced in the years to come. They have been modified to prevent them forming large complex molecules when injected under the skin (a process that occurs to a varying extent with other insulins), thus speeding up their absorption and action. Their big potential advantage is – at least for Humalog and NovoRapid – that they don't need to be injected until immediately before the meal, and their action more closely matches the digestion of the meal than that of conventional clear insulins. This results in better control of the rise in blood glucose following meal digestion and absorption with lowering of the peak glucose concentration. They have another advantage, stemming from their short action: when injected before breakfast, they are less likely to cause hypos before lunch as their effects wear off more quickly. They are ideally suited for the popular 'basal plus bolus' regimens, that is, a long-acting 'basal' insulin at night with a 'bolus' of short-acting insulin before each meal, and are available in cartridges and disposable pens.

I have been having hypos at night and my doctor is keen to change my background insulin to a new long-acting insulin, which he says will solve the problem. How will this help?

He would probably like you to try one of the new insulin analogues. These last longer than your present insulin which is likely to be a form of isophane insulin. This was developed in Denmark 60 years ago and has been the standard background insulin for the past 20 years. Isophane has the drawback that it only lasts for 12 to 16 hours and has a very variable absorption pattern. This means that even if you take identical doses of isophane on consecutive nights, the rate of absorption may vary greatly. This explains why you can wake with a glucose level of 7 one morning and 17 the next. The two new long-acting insulins have been designed to enter the bloodstream slowly and to last for up to 24 hours. Lantus® (glargine) has the longer action and lasts for 24 hours in many people. Levemir® (detemir) probably has a shorter duration of action than Lantus, but is said to have a more consistent action than other long-acting insulins. Most people who change from isophane to Lantus or Levemir get on well with the new insulin and find that their dose of background insulin is more effective and predictable.

My practice nurse would like me to try a new long-acting insulin but tells me there are two options and she is not sure which one to use in my case. Could you please elaborate?

There are two long-acting analogue insulins: detemir (Levemir®) and glargine (Lantus®). They are both 'designer' insulins which are intended to last for up to 24 hours. There is not much to choose between them. Detemir is probably more consistent in its action and glargine has a slightly longer duration of action. This means that as a background insulin, you are more likely to have to take detemir twice a day – usually before breakfast and at bedtime. Glargine is in a slightly acid solution and some people complain that it stings a little when injected.

For the past four years, I have used Actrapid insulin before meals and Insulatard at bedtime. I've recently been changed to NovoRapid as mealtime insulin and I'm not very happy. My control has got worse and I seem to need much larger doses of NovoRapid compared with the dose of Actrapid. It is very disheartening as I was told the new insulin would make life easier.

This is a common problem with changing to NovoRapid and there is a simple explanation. It concerns the need for background insulin 24 hours a day. Actrapid is a longer-acting insulin than NovoRapid and usually lasts from one meal to the next. Thus Actrapid before a meal provides the surge of insulin for the meal but once you are back in the basal (unfed) state, the activity of Actrapid persists, acting as background insulin until your next insulin injection. This has the downside of putting you at risk of a hypo before your next meal and increasing the need for snacks between meals. NovoRapid (exactly like Humalog) is designed to act more rapidly and wear off sooner than Actrapid. The risk of hypo is reduced but now there are times between meals when you have no background insulin.

There are two solutions to this problem. One is to take an extra injection of Insulatard before breakfast. This would last throughout the day until your second injection of Insulatard at bedtime. The other option is to change to a longer-acting analogue such as glargine or detemir. These last for up to 24 hours, unlike Insulatard which only has a duration of 16 hours. Whoever replaced your Actrapid with NovoRapid should have predicted this need to change your background insulin.

What should I do if I suddenly realise I have missed an injection?

It is quite easy to forget to give yourself an injection or – even worse – to be unable to remember whether or not you have had your injection. If this happens you should measure your blood glucose level to help you decide what to do next.

If your blood glucose is high (more than 10 mmol/L) you probably did forget your injection and you should have some short-acting insulin as soon as possible. The dose depends on how close you are to the next injection time. If your blood glucose is normal or low (7 mmol/L or less) you probably did have your injection even if you have forgotten doing it. It would be safest to check your blood glucose again before your next meal and, if it is high, to have an extra dose of short-acting insulin.

Does the timing of the injections matter? Can a person who is on two injections a day take them at 10 a.m. and 4 p.m.?

Unless you are taking Humalog or NovoRapid, which are very quick-acting insulins and should be taken just before a meal, it is best to have your insulin about 30 minutes before a meal, and we discuss this further in the next section *Diet and insulin*. If you have your main meals in the middle of the morning and in the afternoon, then you could try giving insulin at the times you suggest. You may find that an afternoon injection may not last the 18 hours until the next morning, which is why most people try to keep their two injections about 12 hours apart.

DOSAGE

I have just left hospital after a heart attack. I was found to have diabetes, which came as an extra bit of bad news. I have been sent home on four injections of insulin a day, but have been told that I may be able to stop insulin after three months. Why was insulin necessary?

In general, once people start insulin, they need to continue this for the rest of their lives. However, you are probably an exception to this rule. A study published in 1995 showed that anyone who had a heart attack *and* a raised blood sugar made a much better recovery if they were treated immediately with insulin while in the coronary care unit and for three months after leaving hospital. This applied to people who were already known to have diabetes and those (like yourself) who were previously undiagnosed. Those patients who received the intensive insulin treatment both in hospital and for another three months had a much smaller risk of having another heart attack over the next 12 months. The exact reason why insulin provides this long-term protection is not understood, but the results of the study have to be taken seriously and acted upon.

In your case it is likely that you will be seen by a diabetes specialist three months after leaving hospital and it should then be possible to stop insulin and try a different treatment for your diabetes. Some patients in your position find that they get on extremely well with insulin and when offered the option of stopping it, they choose to continue on the grounds that at some stage in the future, they are likely to need insulin again and they cannot see the point of stopping it for a few years.

Is my insulin requirement likely to vary at different times of the year because of the weather?

Several people have remarked that their dose of insulin needs to be altered in very hot weather: some need to give themselves more insulin and others less. This is probably because people react in different ways to a heatwave. There is a tendency to eat less and take less exercise in tropical conditions. However, because blood flow to the skin is increased in warm temperatures, this could speed up the absorption of the injected insulin and mean that a given dose will not last as long. Everyone is different and you will have to find out for yourself how hot weather affects your own blood glucose.

If my insulin requirements decrease over the years, does this mean that the pancreas has gradually started to produce more natural insulin than when I was younger?

No. It is most unlikely that after many years of diabetes your pancreas will start to produce natural insulin. However, this reduction in dose in older people is well recognised. It could be that you were having more insulin than you really needed in the past. Since the introduction of blood glucose measurement many people are found to be having too much insulin, or sometimes too much at one time of the day and not enough at another. Other possible explanations for older people needing less insulin are that they eat less food, they become thinner, they have a different exercise pattern, and there may be hormonal changes.

INJECTING

Insulin pens

What is an insulin pen, and what are the advantages of using one?

An insulin pen consists of a cartridge of insulin inside a case like a fountain pen which is used with a special disposable needle. After dialling the required number of units of insulin and inserting the needle into the skin, you press the plunger or button and the pen will release the correct dose of insulin. There are also pens which have insulin built in and these are known as prefilled pens, preloaded or disposable pens. All cartridges and prefilled pens now contain 300 units of insulin and are likely to last several days before needing to be changed. Available pens are listed in Table 3.2. In general the pens are only compatible with insulin cartridges from the same manufacturer.

The great advantage of insulin pens is that they are easier to use than syringe and needle and more convenient. It is simple to give an injection away from home, for example at work, in a restaurant or when travelling. If your eyesight is not good you may find the dial-a-dose clicking sound helps to reassure you that you have dialled up the correct dose. Some pens give a distinct click with each unit or two units dialled.

If you suffer from arthritis or nerve damage in your hands you are likelier to find a pen easier to use than drawing up insulin in a conventional syringe. All these pens rely on ordinary finger pressure for the injection, that is, they are not automatic injectors, but some may be easier than others. For example, the InnoLet® prefilled pen has been especially designed to have a distinctive click and needs mild finger pressure to inject the insulin.

If you find it difficult to inject your insulin because of fear of needles, but would like to use a pen, Novo Nordisk has introduced the PenMate® which hides the needle from view when the injection is given. The PenMate can be obtained on prescription.

Table 3.2 Insulin pens

Company	Pen name	Increments	Dosage range	Insulin used in pen	Reusable or prefilled
Owen Mumford	Autopen Classic	1 unit	1–21	Insulin from Lilly or Wockhardt	Reusable
	Autopen Classic	2 units	2–42	Insulin from Lilly or Wockhardt	Reusable
	Autopen 24	1 unit	1–21	Glargine insulin (Lantus*)	Reusable
	Autopen 24	2 units	2–42	Glargine insulin (Lantus*)	Reusable
Novo Nordisk	Novopen 3 Classic	1 unit	1–70	Any Novo Nordisk insulin	Reusable
	Novopen 3 Fun	1 unit	1–70	Any Novo Nordisk insulin	Reusable
	Novopen Junior	½ unit	1–35	Any Novo Nordisk insulin	Reusable
	Innolet	1 unit	1–50	Mixtard* 30 and Insulatard	Prefilled
	Flexpen	1 unit	1–60	NovoRapid*, Levemir* and Novomix 30	Prefilled
Prefilled					
Lilly	Humapen Luxura	1 unit	1–60	Any Lilly insulin	Reusable
	Humapen Ergo	1 unit	1–60	Any Lilly insulin	Reusable
	Lilly Prefilled Pen	1 unit	1–60	Humalog* Mix50, Humalog* Mix25, Humalog, Humulin I and Humulin M3*	Prefilled
Sanofi-Aventis	OptiClik	1 unit	1–80	Glargine insulin (Lantus*)	Reusable
	Optiset	2 units	2–40	Glargine insulin (Lantus*)	Prefilled
	Optipen Pro	1 unit	1–60	Any Sanofi-Aventis insulin	Reusable

Several makes of pen are available and your healthcare professional will show you the current models. Insulin pens are now available on prescription except for the OptiClik Pen which can be obtained from your nurse. In an urgent situation most pens are available from your hospital diabetic clinic. It may help to have two pens so one can be used as a back-up in case of breakage or loss.

Addresses for all the companies mentioned here can be found in Appendix 2.

I have been told I need four injections a day. I am worried that I might get the insulins mixed up. What can I do to prevent this?

Many people now take three, four or five insulin injections a day and this will mean using two or even three different types of insulin. This is known as a 'basal bolus' or multiple injection regimen. The 'basal' insulin is the long-acting background insulin and the 'bolus' dose is taken when a meal or a large snack is eaten. Some people may take a fixed mixture of insulin in the morning, a fast-acting insulin with their evening meal and a background insulin at bedtime.

The idea of using a multiple injection regimen is to try to mimic the normal insulin secretion of the pancreas, by giving small doses of short-acting insulin to cover meals and a longer-acting insulin once a day to act as a background insulin. The insulin pen was originally developed to make it more convenient for people to inject four times a day. We agree that it can be confusing if you are taking two or three insulins but most pens are available in different colours to help distinguish the different insulins being used. If you are using prefilled pens, these are already colour-coded.

Some people whose lifestyle means they eat at irregular times find their diabetes much more manageable with a basal bolus regimen. There is more flexibility over the timing of meals, as the insulin is not taken until just before the meal is eaten. In practice some people may also need some long-acting insulin taken in the morning to 'top up' the evening background insulin but this will depend on the type of insulin used.

Injectors

What is the 'jet' injector?

This is a needle-free injector, which works by penetrating the skin with insulin using very high pressure jets. It is not entirely painless and is fairly bulky. The recent model available in the UK (MHI-500) has been superceded by a new model, SQ-PEN; see the website www.SQ-PEN.com for details.

Practical aspects of pens, needles, syringes and bottles

When I was discharged from hospital with newly-diagnosed diabetes I was given a pen device and a few disposable syringes and needles for my injections. How do I obtain more?

Pen devices, disposable insulin syringes and pen needles are available free on prescription. Your GP will supply you with a prescription for any make of insulin syringe and/or insulin pen needles that you choose, and they can then be obtained without charge from a chemist.

Alternatively you can buy them at your own cost directly from the chemist without a prescription, or you can send for them by post from suppliers such as Owen Mumford (Medical Shop). Their address is in Appendix 2.

What is the best way of disposing of insulin syringes and pen needles?

There is a device available called the BD Safe-Clip® which cuts the needle off the top of a syringe or insulin pen and retains it in the device. Once the needle is clipped off, put the used syringe or pen needle hub into a rigid sealable container (available on prescription as a Sharps bin) along with your lancets and follow your local council guidelines for safe disposal of medical waste. Some local authorities provide special containers and a collection service for people who are treated with insulin; however, there is no national policy.

The BD Safe-Clip is available free on prescription from your GP.

I have heard that pen needles and disposable syringes can be reused. How many times can they be reused and how can they be kept clean in between injections?

While pen needles and disposable syringes are designed to be used only once, some people do reuse them. However, reusing needles causes them to become blunt, and they can bend very easily. The tiny point on the end can also break off and remain embedded in the flesh. Needles have a fine coating of lubricant on them so they glide in and out of the skin, and reusing them removes this lubricant and may cause a more painful injection. So there are many reasons to use each needle once only.

If you decide to reuse them make sure the protective cover is placed over the needle.

There is a bewildering array of syringes and needles on the market. Which are the best types to use?

In the UK we use three sizes of syringe. They are used with U100 insulin, which is the standard strength of insulin in the UK and most countries, containing 100 units of insulin per 1 millilitre.

- The 0.5 mL syringe. This is marked with 50 single divisions for taking not more than 50 units of insulin in one injection.

- The 1 mL syringe, marked up to 100 units in 2 unit divisions for those taking more than 50 units of insulin in one injection.

- The 0.3 mL syringe, designed for children or those taking less than 30 units of insulin in one injection.

The most popular make is the BD syringe which comes complete with a fixed Micro-Fine+ 12.7 mm needle, but there are several other makes available.

All these syringes are marked with the word INSULIN on the side of the syringe and graduated in units of insulin. No other type should be used to inject insulin. They are all shown in Figure 3.2.

What length of needle should I use on my insulin pen?

There are several lengths of needle available today ranging from 5 mm to 12.7 mm. As a rule, they are used as follows:

- the 5 or 6 mm needle for children and thin to normal weight adults without a lifted skin fold (this means injecting straight into the skin without pinching it first);

- the 8 mm for normal weight adults with a lifted skin fold (loosely pinched);

- the 12 or 12.7 mm needle for overweight adults also with a lifted skin fold.

Ask your healthcare professional for the needle length and injection technique the most appropriate for you.

I am partially sighted. What pens or syringes are available for people like me, or for people who are blind? Are there any gadgets that would help me with my injections?

Most visually impaired people are advised to use an insulin pen rather than a syringe because you do not need to draw up insulin or check for air bubbles. The dialling mechanism usually has a distinctive clicking sound which reassures you that you have taken the correct dose. It is quite easy to use once the technique has been mastered, and offers a good choice of different types of insulin. This should be discussed with your physician or diabetes specialist nurse. There is a section *Insulin pens* earlier in this chapter.

Novo Nordisk produces a device called Innolet® that might well suit you. It is a disposable insulin pen with a large clock-like dial and a loud clicking sound with each unit dialled. It has raised spots at every 5 units marked. It also has a 'rocker' that allows you to rest the device on your skin before moving the needle forward to inject. It is easier to hold as it has a large grip.

Figure 3.2 Insulin syringes: 0.3 mL, 0.5 mL and 1 mL

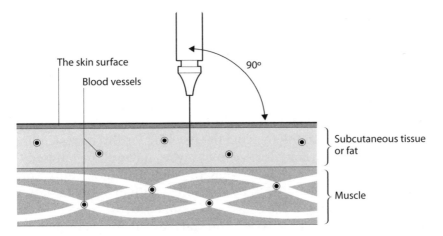

The skin surface

Blood vessels

90°

Subcutaneous tissue or fat

Muscle

Figure 3.3 Skin layers

Where should I keep my supplies of insulin?

Stores of insulin should ideally be kept in a refrigerator, but not in the freezer or freezing compartment. The ideal storage temperature is between 2° and 8°C. Below 0°C insulin is destroyed, and from 30°C upwards, insulin activity progressively decreases. If you do not have a fridge, then insulin may be stored for about a month at room temperature but keep it away from sources of direct heat such as radiators and strong sunlight. Many people prefer to keep their insulin bottle and/or their insulin pen that is in current use at room temperature as it may make the injection more comfortable (cold insulin increases the pain of the injection).

Should I wipe the top of the insulin bottle or insulin cartridge with spirit before use?

It is generally accepted that it is not necessary to clean the cartridge or insulin bottle top before use.

DIET AND INSULIN

I have been told that I am going to have to start insulin after many years of diet and tablets. Will my diet need to change?

It would be helpful if you could discuss your present eating habits and lifestyle with a dietitian before you start on insulin. If you have been trying to avoid the need for insulin by restricting the amount of carbohydrate you eat, you may well be advised to regulate your intake to balance with your insulin. Because your diabetes is no longer able to be controlled with diet and tablets, it is very likely that you are passing out some glucose in your urine. This is a loss of calories. When you start insulin and your diabetes becomes more controlled this loss of glucose in your urine should stop and your weight may increase. Therefore this would be an excellent opportunity to discuss any possible changes with a dietitian.

I am quite a thin person but have been told to watch my 'diet'. Why?

The word 'diet' can often be misleading, as many people think of a diet only in terms of a weight-reducing diet. But 'diet' just means our food intake, or it can mean a course of food prescribed for a particular disorder. For a person with diabetes your diet is your eating plan. It might be less confusing if we said 'food plan' or 'eating plan' instead, but most of us use 'diet' in our everyday conversation as it is a familiar term.

Everyone with diabetes, regardless of their weight, should be encouraged to follow a healthy eating plan or diet. If you are taking insulin then the aim is to balance your food, activity and insulin.

Advice would include the following points.

- Eat some carbohydrate foods at each meal. Carbohydrate foods are starchy or sugary foods such as bread, pasta, potatoes, rice, chapatti, roti, pulses, cereals, fruit, biscuits and crackers.

- Eat only moderate amounts of proteins, even though they are an essential part of everyone's food intake. Foods high in proteins include meat, fish, eggs, cheese, pulses including soya products, Quorn and nuts.

- Be careful with fats. Fats are used for energy and are a more concentrated source of calories than either carbohydrate or protein. Taken in excess, fats can lead to weight gain. Examples of fats are butter, margarine, cream, lard, ghee and vegetable oils. Fried food, cakes and pastries are also high in fats. The choice of fats can also be important as saturated fats and trans-fats can increase your risk of heart disease, so choosing more monounsaturated fats, such as olive oil, is recommended.

Most people eat roughly the same amount of food each day so keeping your carbohydrate and calorie intake fairly constant both in quantity and timing can help when finding a balance with your insulin. Both food and insulin may have to be adjusted for exercise. A dietitian can assess your diet and advise you on the essential changes you need to make while trying to retain as much as possible of your previous eating pattern.

I understand that different forms of carbohydrate have different rates of digestion and that this affects the rise in blood glucose after a meal. I gather there is a 'glycaemic index' for each type of carbohydrate. What is this glycaemic index?

The glycaemic index (GI) is a measure of how quickly foods that contain carbohydrate raise blood glucose levels. Each food is given a number relating to its effect on blood glucose. Foods with a high GI are quickly converted to glucose when eaten and cause a sharp rise in blood glucose levels. Foods with a low GI are converted to glucose much more slowly and produce a more gradual rise in blood glucose. The GI only tells us how quickly a food raises blood glucose when it is eaten on its own and as we usually eat a combination of foods this can change the overall GI of a meal. We do not recommend cutting out all foods with a high GI because your diet needs to be appealing as well as balanced. Low GI foods are generally more filling and can help control hunger as well as blood glucose levels, so they may help with weight loss. You need to be aware that the portion of carbohydrate is also important so eating large quantities of low GI foods can still affect your overall control. Some low GI foods, such as crisps and chocolate, are higher in fat and calories, so choices have to be made sensibly.

Knowing which foods have a high GI can be helpful for treating hypos as these will raise blood glucose more quickly. Table 3.3 gives the GI of some popular foods. The website www.glycaemicindex.com will give you more information on glycaemic index.

How long before eating should I have my insulin injection?

The answer depends on the speed of onset of the insulin you are using.

If you are taking one of the fast-acting analogue insulins such as Humalog® or NovoRapid®, this should normally be injected just before a meal. However, some people prefer to inject immediately after the meal, when they know exactly how much they have eaten.

The older short-acting insulins, such as Actrapid and Humulin S, take longer to have their effect and ideally should be taken 30 minutes before your meal. If your pre-meal blood glucose is low you should delay your injection until you are ready to eat.

I am on two injections a day. Sometimes I find it inconvenient to take my evening injection. Can I skip it and have a meal containing no carbohydrate?

It would not be a good idea to skip your second (evening) injection, as this would leave you without insulin cover overnight. As the effect of your morning injection wears off, your blood glucose levels will rise even if you have eaten no carbohydrate. Insulin pens are easy to carry and should make it relatively easy to inject in most situations. If you need more flexibility in your insulin regimen then speak to your diabetes specialist nurse, who could explain alternative regimens for you to consider.

Do people taking insulin need to eat snacks in between meals?

Sometimes they do. When the pancreas functions normally, it produces insulin 'on demand' when you eat and 'switches off' when the food has been used up. Injected insulin does not 'switch off' in this way. As injected insulin has a peak effect at certain times of the day, it is important for you to cover its action by eating a certain amount of carbohydrates, or you will have a hypo. It is worth remembering that the carbohydrates will last longer if they have a lower glycaemic index (usually rich in fibre), as they are more slowly absorbed (see Table 3.3).

If you are taking a normal insulin before meals, you could try a very short-acting insulin analogue, such as NovoRapid® or Humalog®. These are designed to provide insulin for the following meal but not to have an effect between meals, so you can avoid snacks. There are many ways in which you can adjust your insulin regimen to suit the life you lead, so talk with your doctor or diabetes specialist nurse about these.

As I have to take insulin should I eat a bedtime snack?

It depends on which insulin regimen you are on and what level your blood glucose is at bedtime. If you are taking mixed insulin twice a day, you may need a *small* bedtime snack, such as a piece of toast, fresh fruit, small sandwich, a small bowl of cereal or a yoghurt. It is not advisable to go to bed with a blood glucose level of less than 7 mmol/litre. If it is lower than this you run the risk of having a hypo during the night. If you are on a regimen of a long-acting insulin and three short-acting insulin injections (basal bolus) a bedtime snack should not be necessary. If you do need a bedtime snack your insulin may need adjusting.

Table 3.3 Glycaemic index – a short table

Different tables may give slightly different results depending on the analysis.

Low GI foods (55 or less)	Medium GI foods (56–69)	High GI foods (70 or more)
All-Bran°, porridge made with water (42), Special K° (54)	muesli (56), Weetabix° (69), Shredded Wheat°	Bran flakes, Rice Krispies°, cornflakes, puffed wheat
multigrain breads, stoneground wholemeal bread (53)	wholemeal bread (69), pitta bread, rye bread	white bread, bagels, French bread, gluten-free bread
lentils, barley, kidney beans, butter beans, baked beans, chickpeas, peas, nuts*		broad beans
sweet potato, crisps (54)*	boiled potatoes	mashed potatoes, jacket potatoes, chips, parsnips
cherries, plums, apples, grapefruit, peaches, kiwi fruit, oranges, grapes, berries, bananas (55), mangos (55)	sultanas, raisins, fruit tinned in syrup ripe bananas	watermelon, dates
wheat pasta, spaghetti, macaroni	basmati rice	white rice, rice pasta
milk, yoghurts, milk chocolate* (49)	ice-cream	jelly beans, jelly babies*

*although these foods have a low GI, it is due to their high fat content and so they are high in calories.
(numbers in brackets give GI of a certain food)

Should I increase my insulin over Christmas to cope with the extra food I shall be eating?

Yes, you can take extra insulin to cover the extra carbohydrates that you eat on any special occasion, not just Christmas. At Christmas most people (including people with diabetes) eat more and this is fine. But it is also worth remembering that extra food will be stored and will increase your weight! Any extra activity (such as a walk, or dancing) will help to reduce the effects of the extra food.

Extra carbohydrate foods will need extra insulin and some trial and error may be required to achieve the correct increase in your dose. It would be safer to increase your insulin by a small amount (e.g. one to two units) at a time, unless you have experience of how much extra you require.

Is it all right for me, as someone who takes insulin, to have a lie in on Sunday or must I get up and have my injection and breakfast at the normal time?

Your insulin treatment needs to fit your chosen lifestyle as much as possible and you should be able have a lie in on a Sunday if you wish! Some trial and error might be necessary and we would encourage you to monitor to see what works for you. If you are on twice-daily insulin and you delay your first injection by several hours, then you may need to reduce this first dose, especially if you are having breakfast and lunch as one meal. If you are taking long-acting insulin first thing in the morning, it may be possible to change the timing of this insulin permanently to allow you the flexibility of lying in when you choose. If you only take short-acting insulin in the morning, it is much easier to omit this insulin and miss breakfast. You should make an appointment with your diabetes nurse to discuss the options of changing your insulin regimen to suit your lifestyle.

I have two injections a day: morning and evening. I keep regular times for breakfast and evening tea but I would like to vary the time that I take lunch. What effect would this have on the control of my diabetes?

As you are taking two injections a day, it is most likely you are on a mixed insulin or a medium-acting insulin. Because insulins have a peak of activity, it is important that you cover this peak with food or you will increase your risk of a hypo. If you are having a later lunch you may have to include a mid-morning snack and be prepared to increase this to avoid a pre-lunch hypo.

Trial and error and careful monitoring will give you the best guide to how much you can alter the timing of your lunch. If you feel you need more flexibility of mealtimes, multiple injections may be a better alternative for you. Your diabetes team can discuss options with you.

Sometimes I suffer from a poor appetite. Is it all right for me to reduce my insulin dose on such occasions?

The answer to this question depends on the number of insulin injections you take each day. If you use basal bolus insulin, it is easy to omit or reduce your mealtime insulin to match your food intake. You should never omit the long-acting dose. If you take insulin twice a day, and your appetite is reduced, you are at risk of a hypo if you miss a meal completely. It is never easy to deal with a variable or erratic meal pattern if you are on premixed insulin, but you could consider reducing the dose, using blood tests to help you decide how much insulin to take. If your appetite continues to be poor, or if you are losing weight unintentionally, you should see a dietitian for advice about food choices when your appetite is poor.

My husband has been putting on weight since being diagnosed as having diabetes three months ago. What are the reasons for this?

Most people lose weight before their diabetes is diagnosed and treated. In uncontrolled diabetes, body fat is broken down and many calories are lost as glucose in the urine (this is discussed in more detail in the section *Symptoms* in Chapter 1). As soon as the diabetes is brought under control, the body fat stops being broken down, the calories are no longer lost and the weight loss stops. Many people, like your husband, begin to put weight back on again.

If he starts to put on too much weight, your husband should discuss this with his diabetes specialist nurse and his dietitian. They will advise him about his diet and activity and, if he is on insulin, about reducing his food intake and insulin simultaneously.

I have been taking insulin for eight years and over this time I have put on a lot of weight. My doctor says that insulin does not make you fat, but if that is so, why have I put on so much weight?

Before starting insulin people often lose weight. This is because when diabetes is not controlled you lose lots of calories as glucose in the urine (see the section *Symptoms* in Chapter 1). When diabetes is controlled, the calories are no longer lost in the urine and the weight loss stops. There is then a tendency for people to put on weight or regain the weight they had lost. Insulin in the correct dose should not make you fat but if you are having too much insulin you have to eat more to prevent hypos. These extra calories will increase your weight. Also initially insulin can increase your appetite, as it lowers your blood glucose.

Trying to lose weight when you are on insulin is possible, but needs to be done slowly, as you cannot make drastic diet changes without upsetting your diabetes control. With careful reduction of both food and insulin, weight loss can be achieved but requires patience and perseverance.

Since I went onto multiple injections to improve my control and fit in with my hectic work schedule I have put on quite a lot of weight. I am really pleased with my control and no longer miss insulin to avoid hypos but why do I keep on getting fatter?

Your change in insulin regimen is helping you control your diabetes and fits in better with your work. It is good that you are not missing your insulin and that there is a better match with your insulin and food intake. Since you are now able to use all the food you eat, any excess you do not need will be stored as fat.

To control your weight you need to balance the food you eat with the amount of energy you use up. Have a careful look at your diet.

Perhaps you are choosing a sensible, healthy diet but your portions are too large.

If you are keen to reduce your weight, start by looking at the amounts of fat and alcohol in your diet, as these are both very concentrated sources of calories. Aim to cut back on any fatty foods, choosing low fat products instead of full fat, and having fruit or a diet yoghurt instead of crisps or biscuits as snacks. Choose lean meat, fish or poultry with the skin removed or Quorn. Include plenty of vegetables. You should aim for a weight loss of between 0.5–1 kg (1–2 lb) a week. If you are not making progress you may have to consider reducing your intake of starchy foods, along with blood glucose monitoring and reduction of your insulin to prevent hypos. Regular exercise will also help use up some of the excess calories. If your weight continues to be a problem, record all your meals and snacks for three or four days and then ask the dietitian to go over them with you to see where further changes can be made.

My partner has diabetes and is trying to lose weight. She eats a low-carbohydrate diet and sticks to this rigidly. I cannot understand why she does not lose any weight.

Reducing a single food group, such as carbohydrate, in her diet will not necessarily lead to a loss of weight. Low carbohydrate diets are often much higher in fats and proteins so the total calories consumed are not necessarily reduced. A better and healthier approach would be to look carefully at what she eats and aim to reduce the higher calorie foods such as fatty foods and alcohol. Avoiding fried foods, using low fat dairy products, taking moderate amounts of protein as low fat meat, fish, chicken or meat substitutes such as tofu or Quorn, increasing fruit and vegetables, choosing carbohydrate foods with a lower glycaemic index, and including some regular activity would be the best long-term plan. Your partner may benefit from help and support from a dietitian or diabetes specialist nurse.

I have heard that there is an anti-obesity pill that works by stopping fat absorption. Would it be suitable for me? I have diabetes and am very overweight.

The tablet you are probably referring to is called Xenical®, the brand name for orlistat. It blocks the digestion of fat and is the first anti-obesity pill not to rely on suppressing appetite. Orlistat manipulates the chemical digestion processes, blocking the action of lipases (enzymes that break up fat in the intestine), so that about 30% of fat in any meal goes undigested. However, there can be unpleasant side effects. The dietary fat that is not absorbed will be rapidly excreted, which can lead to stomach cramps, diarrhoea and 'oily spotting'. Orlistat is recommended for people with diabetes and if you manage to lose weight, it will help your diabetic control. The company has a very useful helpline which provides a whole package of advice about lifestyle. People who make use of the helpline are much more likely to succeed with Orlistat.

HYPOS

Since my wife has been started on insulin she has had funny turns. What is the cause of this?

Your wife's funny turns are likely to be due to a low blood glucose level. The medical term is hypoglycaemia that most people call 'hypo' for short. When the blood glucose falls below a certain level (usually 3 mmol/litre), the brain is affected. Highly dependent on glucose, the brain stops working properly and begins to produce symptoms such as weakness of the legs, double or blurred vision, confusion, headache and, in severe cases, loss of consciousness and convulsions. Hypoglycaemia will also trigger the production of adrenaline, a hormone responsible for causing sweating, rapid heartbeat and feelings of panic and anxiety. Children often describe a 'dizzy feeling' or just 'tiredness' when they are hypoglycaemic. Most people find it hard to describe how they feel when hypo but the proof is that the blood glucose is low. If there is any doubt about the accuracy of your meter readings, it is always safer to take glucose or sugar if you're feeling odd. Symptoms of hypoglycaemia are shown in Table 3.4.

What is the best thing to take when I have a hypo?

This very much depends at which stage you recognise the hypo is developing. In the early stages the best treatment would be to have a meal or snack if one is due, or if there is some time before your next meal, an extra snack such as fruit, a sandwich or biscuits.

If your hypo is fairly well advanced, you need to take some very rapidly-absorbed carbohydrates. This is best taken as sugar, sweets or fruit juice or, for even greater speed, a sugary drink such as ordinary (not 'diet') Coke, lemonade or Lucozade. Good things to carry in your pocket are also glucose tablets such as Dextro-Energy as they are absorbed very quickly (three tablets of Dextro-Energy contain 10 g of glucose). They are also less likely to be eaten when you are not hypo than ordinary sweets!

You should eat some bread, biscuits or a small sandwich after the sugar or sugary drink.

I am taking soluble and isophane insulin twice a day and am getting hypos two to three hours after my evening meal. As I live alone this has been worrying me. What can I do?

Anyone who is having frequent hypos at a particular time of day can easily put this right by adjusting their insulin dose. In this case, you are having hypos at the time when your evening dose of soluble insulin is working. You should reduce the amount of soluble insulin you take in the evening until you have stopped having hypos at that time. On the other hand, hypos before your evening meal could be corrected by reducing your morning dose of intermediate-acting (isophane) insulin.

Table 3.4 Symptoms of a 'hypo'

Cause	Symptom
Adrenaline response	Sweating
	Pounding heart
	Shaking/trembling
	Hunger
	Anxiousness
	Tingling
Brain's lack of glucose	Confusion/difficulty in thinking
	Drowsiness/weakness
	Odd ('stroppy') behaviour
	Speech difficulty
Non-specific	Nausea
	Headache
	Tiredness

I have recently lost my warning signs for hypos. Is it likely that they will return?

Very tight diabetic control is known to reduce hypoglycaemic awareness. A study carried out with the help of people who had lost their warning symptoms showed that when the participants kept their blood sugar above 4 mmol/L continuously for three months, avoiding hypos altogether, they experienced partial or complete restoration of warning symptoms. Do you think that your diabetes could be too tightly controlled? If so, it may be worth discussing this with your diabetes team and reducing your dose of insulin.

My father has had diabetes for 20 years. Recently he had what his doctor calls epileptic fits. Would you tell me how to help him and if there is a cure?

A bad hypo may bring on a fit and it is important to check your father's blood glucose during an attack. If the glucose level is low, reducing his insulin should stop the fits. If the fits are not due to a low blood glucose level, it should be possible to control them by making sure he takes his epilepsy tablets regularly – ask his doctor for more details about these.

Can insulin reactions eventually cause permanent brain damage?

Many people ask about this as it is a great source of anxiety. The brain recovers quickly from a hypo and there is unlikely to be permanent damage, even after a severe attack with convulsions. Very prolonged hypoglycaemia can occur in someone with a tumour that produces insulin, and if a person is unconscious for days on end then the brain will not recover completely. This is not likely to occur in people with diabetes, in whom the insulin wears off after a few hours. However, there is some evidence that people who have very frequent hypos over many years may be at greater risk of dementia in later life.

If someone on insulin becomes very depressed, would they be able to commit suicide by taking an overdose of insulin?

Without dealing with the moral aspect of this question, we would strongly advise anyone against trying to commit suicide using insulin. It may sometimes lead to a painless death by hypoglycaemia but we know several cases where the person in question has lowered their blood sugar to dangerous levels for enough time to cause permanent brain damage but not to the level where it will lead to death. Most long-term brain injury units have one or two patients who are there because of a failed attempt to end their lives using insulin and this is a very sad situation for both the person concerned and for those close to them.

I have heard that there is an opposite to insulin called glucagon. Is this something like glucose and can it be used to bring someone round from a hypo?

G lucagon is a hormone which, like insulin, is produced by the pancreas. It causes glucose to be released into the bloodstream from stores of starch in the liver. Glucagon can also be injected to bring someone round from a hypo if they are unconscious or too restless to swallow glucose. Glucagon cannot be stored in solution like insulin. It comes in a kit containing a vial with glucagon powder plus a syringe and sterile fluid for dissolving the powder. The process of dissolving the glucagon and drawing it into the syringe may be difficult, especially if you are feeling panicky. It is worth asking the diabetes nurse to show you and your likely helper how to draw up glucagon.

Glucagon only has a short-lasting effect and it is therefore important to follow it up with some sugar by mouth to prevent a relapse of coma. When children have a glucagon injection their blood glucose level may rise sharply and make them feel sick, so they won't want more sugar. It is best to do a blood test to help decide whether more glucose is really needed immediately. More sustaining carbohydrates (such as bread or biscuits) should be given as soon as they feel well enough to eat, as the blood glucose level can fall again later.

When I gave my wife a glucagon injection recently, she vomited. Is this normal?

S ome people do vomit when regaining consciousness after a glucagon injection, particularly children. If only half the content of the vial is given (0.5 mg), it will usually be enough to correct the hypo, but less likely to cause sickness.

My diabetes was controlled by tablets for 20 years but two years ago my doctor recommended that I begin insulin treatment. I am well controlled but my sleep is often disturbed by dreams, or I wake up feeling hungry. Can you advise me what to do if this happens?

You may be going hypo during the night. It has been shown that many people have a low blood glucose in the early hours and, provided that they feel all right and sleep well, this probably does not matter. However, if you are regularly waking up with hypo symptoms (such as hunger) or having nightmares, you should first check whether you are hypo by measuring your blood glucose level at around 3 a.m. when it is usually the lowest. If the reading is below 4 mmol/L you need to reduce your evening dose of intermediate-acting insulin. If your blood glucose is then high before breakfast the next day, an injection of intermediate-acting insulin taken before going to bed instead of before your evening meal may solve your problem.

Am I correct in thinking that only people on insulin can have hypos?

No. Some of the tablets used for treating Type 2 diabetes can also cause hypos. The commonly used ones are glibenclamide (Euglucon®, Daonil®) and gliclazide (Diamicron®). These hypos will improve with glucose in the normal way but, because the tablets have a longer action than insulin, the hypo may return again after several hours. Anyone having hypos on tablets probably needs to reduce the dose. Metformin and the glitazones, however, do not cause hypos.

4 | Monitoring and control

The key to a successful life with diabetes is achieving good blood glucose control. Your degree of success can be judged only by measurements of your body's response to treatment. If you have diabetes, the fact that you feel well does not necessarily mean that your blood glucose is well controlled. It is only when control goes badly wrong that you may be aware that something is amiss. If your blood glucose is too low, you may be aware of hypo symptoms – if left untreated this may progress to unconsciousness (hypoglycaemic coma). At the other end of the spectrum, when the blood glucose concentration rises very steeply, you may be aware of increased thirst and passing urine excessively – left untreated, this may progress to nausea, vomiting, weakness, and eventual clouding of consciousness and coma (a condition called ketoacidosis). It has long been apparent that relying on how you feel is too imprecise, even though some people may be able to 'feel' subtle changes in their control. For this reason, many different tests have been developed to allow precise measurement of control and, as the years go by, these tests become more efficient and accurate.

The involvement of the person with diabetes in monitoring and control of their own condition has always been essential for successful treatment. With the development of blood glucose monitoring, this has become even more apparent: it allows you to measure precisely how effective you are at balancing the conflicting forces of diet, exercise and insulin, and to make adjustments in order to maintain this balance. In the early days after the discovery of insulin, urine tests were the only tests available and it required a small laboratory even to do these. Urine tests have always had the disadvantage that they are only an indirect indicator of what you really need to know, which is the level of glucose in the blood. Blood glucose monitoring first became available to people with diabetes in 1977 and is now widely accepted. As anyone who has monitored glucose levels in the blood will know, these vary considerably throughout the day as well as from day to day. For this reason, a single reading at a twice yearly visit to the local diabetes clinic is of limited value in assessing long-term success or failure with control.

The introduction of haemoglobin A_{1c} (glycosylated haemoglobin or HbA_{1c}) has provided a very reliable test for longer-term monitoring of average blood glucose levels (taking into account the peaks and troughs) over an interval of two to three months. Someone with diabetes should aim at a target HbA_{1c} of 7%, which indicates that the blood glucose has been contained within the near normal range. Provided there have been no troublesome hypoglycaemic attacks, this means that balance of diabetes has been excellent and no further changes are required. Achieving a normal HbA_{1c} level and maintaining it as near normal as possible is an important goal. Not everyone can achieve this, but it is undoubtedly the most effective way of eliminating the risk of long-term complications.

This has been shown for Type 2 diabetes by the UK Prospective Diabetes Study. This major research project took place over twenty years in 23 centres in England, Scotland and Northern Ireland. Over 5000 patients with newly diagnosed Type 2 diabetes took part and the results showed that keeping the HbA_{1c} down to 7% reduced the risk of all complications of diabetes. For more details see the question which follows.

Diabetes care in the UK has been set new standards by the government in the form of a National Service Framework (NSF) for care in England, Wales and Northern Ireland and SIGN (Scottish Intercollegiate Guidelines Network) in Scotland. The NSF is a complex project which will not reach its final goal until 2013. However, it is good that the government is putting pressure on healthcare providers to achieve certain standards. Details of the NSF can be found on p. 140.

WHY MONITOR?

I developed diabetes at the age of 56 and am struggling to control my sugars with tablets. However, I feel perfectly well and wonder why my doctor is so keen for me to have good control.

Until 1998, there was some doubt about the need for tight control of blood glucose in Type 2 diabetes, which is the most common sort of diabetes developing later in life. The results of a large British research project – the UK Prospective Diabetes Study (UKPDS) – were then published, and provided clear evidence that the risk of complications in Type 2 diabetes was higher in those people with higher levels of blood glucose and thus of HbA_{1c}. The 5000 people with diabetes in the study were randomly divided into two groups, one with tight control and the other with higher blood sugars. The group with tighter control had 25% less eye disease and 16% less risk of a heart attack.

The study confirmed that in most people Type 2 diabetes gets steadily worse with time. Thus people who are initially well controlled on tablets, usually need insulin a few years later. The UKPDS also showed that people with Type 2 diabetes benefit from a very strict control of blood pressure, which reduces the risks of heart disease, strokes and eye problems. When the UKPDS was closed in 1997, those patients who took part were followed up for another 10 years and the results were published in 2008. These results showed that when the study came to an end the difference in blood glucose control between the two groups was lost and all patients had the same level of control over the next 10 years. Despite this, patients who had tight control in the years immediately following diagnosis had lower risks of diabetic complications, including heart attack, and this reduction in risk was maintained for the next 10 years. The message is that good blood glucose control in the early years leads to extended benefits and so there should be no delay before starting treatment.

I have Type 2 diabetes and am treated with insulin. I am not very keen on testing my blood and sometimes feel guilty about this. How often do I really need to test?

When you first went on insulin you probably had support from family and workmates and close contact with a practice nurse. It can be depressing when the initial interest fades and you have to come to terms with the fact that the routine of diabetes will never go away. This is a time when people may stop doing regular blood tests. We have interviewed a number of people who have given up testing and these are the most common reasons they give.

- Testing is messy and bloody.
- I haven't got time/can't be bothered to test my blood.
- There is no need to test if you feel all right.
- Testing my blood brings it home to me that I have diabetes.

- It is inconvenient/embarrassing to test in public or at work.

- Insulin injections are essential, blood tests are not.

- A bad test makes me feel even more depressed about my diabetes.

- There is no point in testing my blood as I don't use the information.

These are the opinions of people living with diabetes and they must be respected. However, we believe that, if you need insulin, you will only achieve good control by doing blood tests since there is no other way of knowing exactly where you are with your diabetes. There is no hard and fast rule about how often you should test and you should be guided by what information you hope to gain from doing a blood test. You should obviously test if it is important to know your glucose level, for example when checking your safety to drive, confirming a hypo or if you feel unwell, or in preparation for exercise. On other occasions, you may simply want to check that your blood sugar level is within the target range. For further guidance, see the advice on blood glucose monitoring on p. 113.

In the past 12 months I have had to increase my insulin dosage several times, but have been unable to get a blood test result that was near normal. I have had diabetes for 25 years and until last year I have always been well controlled. What has gone wrong?

Here are a few reasons why your blood glucose levels may have crept up and why you need more insulin after many years of good control:

- less exercise, meaning that more insulin is needed for your food intake;

- an increase in the amount of food you eat;

- increased stress or emotional upsets;

- any illness that lingers on, leading to a need for more insulin;

- technical problems with injections such as the appearance of lumps from repeated doses of insulin into the same site;

- increase in weight and middle-age spread;

- treatment with certain drugs, especially steroids.

Apart from these identified reasons, some people do find that the dose of insulin that they need may vary by quite large amounts with no obvious explanation.

Can stress influence blood glucose readings?

Yes, but the response varies from one person to another. In some people stress tends to make the blood glucose rise whereas in other people it may increase the risk of hypoglycaemia.

MONITORING IN TYPE 2 DIABETES

My GP says blood tests are very expensive and wants me to cut down the number of tests. I take metformin and gliclazide to control my diabetes. How often should I be testing?

There is great pressure on GPs to reduce their spending on drugs and since blood glucose testing strips are very expensive, these are often selected as a target for cutting costs. Most strips cost up to £28 for 50. It is a sad fact that some people with diabetes test their blood sugars very frequently and do not make use of the results. People on tablets for diabetes certainly do not need to test as frequently as those taking insulin, but there are important and valid reasons for you needing to have the ability to check your blood sugar.

First, it is useful to take a typical day and test a number of times at random to find the range of your blood sugars. You may find that two hours after a meal your sugars climb well into the teens. Then, if you have a questioning mind, you will want to discover which foods are responsible. Thus blood glucose monitoring is a powerful educational tool, which can help you discover the effect of different foodstuffs. Our local Primary Care Trusts, which are responsible for advising GPs about economical prescribing, have agreed blood glucose monitoring guidelines which appear in Figure 4.2. They suggest that you test your blood between twice a week and twice a day, depending on the type of treatment you take. As long as you are obtaining useful information, which you will act on, you should continue testing your blood sugar.

BLOOD GLUCOSE TESTING

What is the normal range of blood glucose in a person who does not have diabetes?

Before meals the range is from 3.5 to 5.5 mmol/litre. After meals it may rise as high as 10 mmol/L depending on the carbohydrate content of the meal. However long a person without diabetes goes without food, the blood glucose concentration never drops below 3 mmol/L, and however much they eat, it never goes above 10 mmol/L.

My blood glucose monitor is calculated in millimoles. What's a millimole?

In the 1960s, international agreement led scientists in most parts of the world to adopt a standard system of metric measurements. The units are called SI units, an abbreviation of their full name – the 'Système International d'Unité'. There are several units, many of which you probably use without thinking about them, such as the metre. The unit for an amount of a substance is called a mole; the prefix 'milli-' means one-thousandth, so a millimole is one-thousandth of a mole. Blood glucose is measured in millimoles of glucose per litre of blood, and this is abbreviated to mmol/L.

Before SI units were introduced, blood glucose was measured in milligrams per 100 millilitres of blood (abbreviated to mg% or to mg per dL) and this measurement is still used in the USA. Table 4.1 shows how one set of units relates to the other.

Is blood glucose monitoring suitable for people whose diabetes is controlled by tablets?

Yes, it is. Everyone with diabetes, whether controlled by diet, diet and tablets, or insulin, should strive for perfect control. Traditionally this has been achieved by regular urine tests at home. Since 1977 there has been a move towards encouraging people to do their own blood glucose measurements. This form of monitoring was first thought to be most suitable for insulin-treated people. However, further experience has shown that it is equally suited to those treated with diet and tablets. The disadvantage of having to prick your finger to obtain a drop of blood is more than compensated for by the

Table 4.1 Blood glucose measurements

1 mmol/L = 18 mg%	2 mmol/L = 36 mg%
3 mmol/L = 54 mg%	4 mmol/L = 72 mg%
5 mmol/L = 90 mg%	6 mmol/L = 108 mg%
7 mmol/L = 126 mg%	8 mmol/L = 144 mg%
9 mmol/L = 162 mg%	10 mmol/L = 180 mg%
12 mmol/L = 216 mg%	15 mmol/L = 270 mg%
20 mmol/L = 360 mg%	22 mmol/L = 396 mg%
25 mmol/L = 450 mg%	30 mmol/L = 540 mg%

increased accuracy and reliability of the readings so obtained. Since blood glucose test strips are expensive, it is important to make use of the test results, either by increasing your knowledge about the effect of different foods or activities (or both) on blood glucose, or by making changes as a result of the information you obtain from the test result. Some GPs tell their patients that blood glucose testing is only necessary for people using insulin. We have agreed some local guidelines about blood testing with our GPs and you will find these in Figure 4.2.

Should I keep my blood glucose monitoring sticks in the fridge with my insulin?

No. It is important to keep them dry as any moisture will affect their activity. The bottle of sticks should be kept in a cool, dry place, and not be exposed to extremely high temperatures. You must put the lid back on the container immediately after removing a strip (unless the strips are individually foil-wrapped). Many of the strips contain enzymes, which are biological substances that do not last forever, and the sticks should never be used beyond their expiry date. If you have any reason to suspect the result of a blood test, it is best to repeat the test using a new bottle of strips.

I had a glucose tolerance test and my highest blood glucose was 17 mmol/L. However, my urine analysis was negative for glucose. Is there a way I could test my blood for glucose without going to the laboratory?

You appear to have a 'high renal threshold' to glucose (see the section *Urine* later in this chapter). This means that it is only at very high concentrations of glucose in the blood that any glucose escapes into your urine. In your case urine tests are unhelpful and blood tests essential. Nowadays most people monitor their blood glucose at home using the compact and convenient meters that are widely available.

There are several different blood testing techniques and most strips can be used only with the meter designed for that strip. Your practice nurse or hospital clinic will be able to show you the various strips and meters that are available and your choice should be made after discussion with them. All the different methods give good results provided that they are used sensibly and after proper instruction. The blood glucose meters are not available on prescription, but the strips are.

There is more information about both strips and meters later in this section, and Table 4.2 lists the meters currently available.

I feel hypo when my blood glucose is normal and only well when it is high. I feel very ill when my doctor tries to keep my blood glucose normal. Am I hooked on a high blood glucose?

When you have had poor control for several years, the brain and other tissues in the body can adjust to a high concentration of glucose in the blood. As a result you may feel hypo at a time when your blood glucose is normal or even high. The long-term outlook for people in your situation is not good unless you can re-educate yourself to tolerate normal blood glucose levels without feeling unwell. This is possible but requires determination and an understanding of the long-term dangers of a high blood glucose.

Your problem can be overcome by regular measurement and a gradual lowering of your blood glucose so that your body has the chance to adjust to the lower levels. You must believe that, however unwell you feel, no harm will be done if your blood glucose remains above 4 mmol/litre. It may take up to six months for this re-education process to take effect, but it will be worth it.

I find that my control is only good for one week a month and that is the week before my period. Why is this and what should I do about it?

In some women the dose of insulin required to control diabetes varies in relation to the menstrual cycle. Your question implies that you become more sensitive to insulin in the week before you menstruate and you probably require more insulin at the other times in your cycle. There is no reason why you should not try to work out a pattern where you reduce your insulin dose in the week before your period and increase it at other times.

The variation is due to different hormones coming from the ovaries during the menstrual cycle. Some of these hormones have an anti-insulin effect. The same sort of effects may occur when a woman is taking oral contraceptive tablets (the Pill) or is pregnant. You should try to make adjustments in the insulin dose in order to compensate for these hormonal changes and to keep the balance of the blood glucose where it should be. Your diabetes clinic doctor or diabetes specialist nurse is the best person to turn to for exact advice on how to make these adjustments.

I have been using Mixtard to control my diabetes for some years. I take 36 units before breakfast and 24 units before my evening meal. My blood tests are normally pretty good except for bedtime when they are often as high as 15 mmol/L. My doctor says my control is not good enough and wants me have more injections each day. What is your view on this?

Twice daily injections of insulin are usually a compromise. It sounds as if your evening dose does not supply enough short-acting insulin to cope with your evening meal, though the long-acting component of Mixtard is able to provide enough overnight background insulin. A fairly simple solution would be to 'split the evening dose'. You would have to take a dose of short-acting insulin before your evening meal and some background insulin at bedtime. The doses would have to be adjusted depending on the results of blood tests. This new arrangement would have the added advantage that you could vary the pre-meal dose of insulin depending on how much you wanted to eat.

Table 4.2 Blood glucose meters

Company	Meter name	Test strip name	Size of sample (in microlitres)	Range of results (in mmoles/L)	Test time (in seconds)
Abbott Diabetes care (helpline 0500 467 466)	Medisense Optium Xceed	Medisense Optium Plus Electrodes (also Medisense B ketone electrodes to measure blood ketone levels)	0.6	1.1–27.8	5
	Freestyle Freedom	Freestyle	0.3	1.1–27.8	5
	Freestyle Mini	Freestyle	0.3	1.1–27.8	7
ADL Healthcare Diagnostics (helpline 0800 08 588 08) truetrack@adlhealthcare.co.uk	TrueTrack SmartSystem	TrueTrack SmartSystem	1.0	1.3–33.3	10
Bayer HealthCare (helpline 0845 600 6030) www.ascensia.co.uk	Ascensia Contour	Ascensia Microfill Test Strips (10 test disc)	0.6	0.6–33.3	15
	Ascensia Breeze	Ascensia Autodisc (10 test disc)	2–3	0.6–33.3	30
CDx Ltd (helpline 0191 564 2036) www.cdx.uk.com	SensoCard Plus (Talking Meter)	SensoCard	0.5	1.1–33.3	5
LifeScan (helpline 0800 121 200) www.lifescan.co.uk	One Touch Ultra	One Touch Ultra Test Strips	1	1.1–33.3	5
	One Touch Ultra Smart	One Touch Ultra Test Strips	1	1.1–33.3	5

Company	Meter name	Test strip name	Size of sample (in microlitres)	Range of results (in mmoles/L)	Test time (in seconds)
Menarini	GlucoMen° Visio	GlucoMen° Visio Sensors	0.8	1.1–33.3	10
(helpline 0800 243 667)	GlucoMen° PC	GlucoMen° sensors	2.0	1.3–33.3	30
visio@menarinidiag.co.uk	GlucoMen° Glyco	GlucoMen° sensors	2.0	1.3–33.3	30
Roche Diagnostics	Accu-chek° Aviva	Accu-chek° Aviva	0.6	0.6–33.3	5
(helpline 0800 701 000)	Accu-chek° Active	Accu-chek° Active Strips	2	0.55–33.3	5
www.accu-chek.co.uk	Compact Plus	Compact Plus	1.5	0.55–33.3	5
	Accu-chek° Advantage	Advantage Plus	4	0.55–33.3	25

Note:

The table above gives a selection of currently available meters. This list is constantly being updated. More extensive lists can be found in the *British National Formulary* (*BNF*) or at www.diabetes.co.uk.

Where is the best place to obtain blood for measuring blood glucose levels?

It is usually easiest to obtain blood from the fingertips. You can use either the pulp, which is the fleshy part of the fingertip, or the sides of the fingertips. The sides of the fingertips are less sensitive than the pulp. Some people like to use the area just below the nailbed. It may be necessary for people such as guitarists, pianists or typists to avoid the finger pulp. There are a couple of meters that allow blood to be taken from the arm (see the question on arm testing later in this chapter).

Which is the best finger pricking device?

All blood lancets (finger prickers) are very similar and there is little to choose between them. The lancets may be used either on their own or in conjunction with an automatic device. They are obtainable on prescription from your GP. Alternatively they can be bought from a chemist, or ordered by post from companies such as Owen Mumford (Medical Shop); see Appendix 2 for addresses.

The automatic devices work on the principle of hiding the lancet from view while piercing the skin very quickly and at a controlled depth. The meter you are using will have had an accompanying finger pricking device. They are not available on prescription, but can be obtained from the manufacturer of your meter (see Table 4.2) or by post from companies such as Owen Mumford (Medical Shop).

Should I clean my fingers with spirit or antiseptic before pricking them?

We do not recommend that you use spirit for cleaning your fingers. Spirit or antiseptic could interfere with the test strip and cause soreness if you have recently pricked the same finger. We suggest that you wash your hands with soap and warm water, or only water, and dry them thoroughly before pricking your finger. The main reason for having a clean finger is to remove any contamination, such as food, that may cause a false blood glucose result.

Will constant finger pricking make my fingers sore?

Y ou may find that your fingers feel sore for the first week or two after starting blood glucose monitoring but this seems to settle down. We have seen many people who have been measuring their blood glucose levels regularly three or four times a day for more than 15 years and who have no problems with sore fingers. The more up-to-date meters use very small amounts of blood and so you don't need to prick your finger too brutally! Don't always use the same finger – try to use different fingers in turn.

Will my fingers take a long time to heal after finger pricking and am I more likely to pick up an infection there?

Y our fingertips should heal as quickly as those of someone without diabetes, but make sure that you are using suitable blood lancets. We have seen only one infected finger among many hundreds of thousands of finger pricks. As long as your hands are clean when you take your blood sample, you should not have any problems.

There are a bewildering number of strips and meters on the market. Which are the best to use?

A few years ago most people were using strips without a meter. This required performing a complicated procedure in order to obtain an accurate blood glucose result. Now in the UK you can only use a strip with a meter. The meters are very similar in terms of reliability and performance. There are small differences, for example the amount of blood required to perform a test or the time it takes for the meter to produce the results (see Table 4.2). Nearly all the meters can be downloaded onto a PC and software is usually available free from the manufacturers.

Blood testing is not just about doing the test but making sense of the results. Your healthcare professional will show you how to use your meter, and you will need further time to discuss your results and what you might need to change in order to achieve the levels you want.

Blood glucose testing strips are available on prescription from your GP. The meters are quite inexpensive and may be available free from your diabetes nurse.

> *I have recently started testing my blood sugar levels but my results do not compare well with the clinic results. What is the reason for this?*

It is not clear if your blood sugar results are being compared with blood sugar tests at the hospital or with another test known as the HbA_{1c}, glycosylated haemoglobin or long-term test. The HbA_{1c} is usually measured only once or twice a year. The test measures the amount of glucose that has attached itself to the red blood cells, throughout their 2–3 month life span (see section *Haemoglobin A_{1c}* later in this chapter). Research tells us that to avoid complications of diabetes the HbA_{1c} should be under 7.5% (see introduction to this chapter). The HbA_{1c} is often described as an average of blood sugar levels but strictly speaking it is not an average. For example, if your HbA_{1c} is 12% your blood sugar levels are likely to be averaging around 19 mmol/L. When you perform a blood sugar test at home you are measuring the result as it is at that minute in time. Two hours later it could be much lower or much higher. The HbA_{1c} is not measuring the highs and lows but what has accumulated in the previous two to three months.

In summary, it is possible that your home blood glucose tests are being compared with the HbA_{1c} which is a different kind of test. Alternatively, the blood is being tested at a different time or on a different blood testing machine, which can cause a variation in results.

I have Type 2 diabetes and have just started tablets. I am
testing my urine but would prefer to test my blood sugar.
Why does my GP not seem keen to prescribe blood testing
strips for me?

Blood glucose monitoring for people with Type 2 diabetes is a controversial area. Some healthcare professionals feel that there is no proof that blood testing helps people improve their diabetic control. Blood testing is reasonably costly and it can be argued that if it doesn't improve things then the expense is not justified. However, you may feel that home blood glucose monitoring may help you to understand your diabetes better. For example, it can tell you what happens if you take exercise or eat a big meal. Blood testing may give you a sense of being more in control. You may wish to discuss with your doctor or nurse how you think you could benefit from testing your blood glucose.

Are the blood glucose meters accurate enough for daily use?

Most results obtained when you are using a meter will be slightly different from the clinic laboratory results or even from different makes of meters because different technological methods are used. These slight differences do not matter and the strips and meters are quite accurate enough for home use provided your technique is correct. If you are concerned that your results may not be accurate you can check the meter yourself by using the quality control solution provided with the meter. Phone the meter company helpline (see Table 4.2) for advice or contact your diabetes specialist nurse who can check both your meter and your technique.

I have heard that there is a watch you can wear that
measures the blood sugar automatically. Is this right?

You are thinking about the GlucoWatch®, developed by a Californian company called Cygnus Inc. Unfortunately there were many technological problems and so the GlucoWatch is currently unavailable in the UK. This device is worn like a wristwatch and measures blood glucose from interstitial fluid every 10–20 minutes depending on the model. The watch had to be fitted with a sensor which only lasted for 12 hours and was expensive to buy.

I have heard that it is now possible to obtain a meter, which can measure the blood glucose constantly without the need for repeated fingerpricks. How do I get hold of one?

Meters which provide a continuous read-out of blood glucose levels are available for research purposes and for short-term use. The eventual aim is to connect these meters to an insulin pump allowing the dose of insulin to be controlled by the level of blood glucose – a true 'artificial pancreas'. The technology is promising but not fully developed.

At present the Minimed Medtronic can record the blood glucose continuously for three days and many diabetes centres will own such a meter. They can be loaned to people who are having problems with their diabetes control and are used to identify patterns of either high or low blood sugars. They do not produce an immediate reading but can be downloaded to a computer to print out a three-day blood glucose curve. Unfortunately the three-day probes are expensive and are not yet practical for long term use.

I have trouble obtaining enough blood to perform a blood sugar test. Is there anything that I can do to make this easier?

The good news is that many of the new meters need only tiny amounts of blood in order to perform a test (see Table 4.2). However, if you are having trouble obtaining enough blood then try warming your hands by washing them in warm water before you start, and drying them thoroughly before pricking your finger. When squeezing the blood out of your finger, try 'milking' the blood out gently, allowing the finger to recover between each squeeze. Do not squeeze so hard that you blanch the finger white.

I am about to buy a meter that allows blood to be taken from the arm. Are there any problems with arm testing?

At the time of writing there are three meters that allow blood for testing to be taken from the arm. They are the OneTouch® Ultra from LifeScan and the FreeStyle® Freedom and Freestyle Mini from Abbott. The OneTouch Ultra and FreeStyle use strips that allow a tiny blood sample to be taken, which makes arm testing feasible. Under certain conditions, samples taken from the arm may differ significantly from fingertip samples, such as when blood glucose is changing rapidly:

- following a meal;
- after an insulin dose;
- when taking physical exercise.

Arm samples should only be used for testing *prior to, or more than two hours after* meals, an insulin dose or physical exercise. Fingertip testing should be used whenever there is a concern about hypoglycaemia (such as before you drive a car), as arm testing may not detect hypoglycaemia. Obtaining sufficient blood from the arm is not always easy but for some it is a welcome alternative to fingertip pricking. Your health professional should be consulted before you begin arm testing.

I have heard that there is a way of obtaining blood from a finger using a laser. Is this true?

The Lasette is a single shot laser that makes a small hole in the finger to obtain a drop of blood, but it is not a blood glucose monitoring device. The use of laser light, as opposed to a steel lancet, reduces tissue damage, and many users of the device report feeling less pain than when using a traditional lancet. It weighs just less than 260 g (9 oz). However, it is very expensive. It is slightly smaller than a videocassette. The Lasette is manufactured by Cell Robotics, and can be obtained from Nutech International, whose address is in Appendix 2.

> *I would like to measure my own blood glucose levels, but as I am now blind I do not know if this is possible. Can it be done?*

After a long spell when no speaking meters were available there is now the new SensoCard® Plus Meter which will speak instructions and also speak the result (see Table 4.2). The meter has recently come down in price. Strips are available on prescription and your pharmacist would need to contact the company, Cobolt Systems Ltd, directly (address in Appendix 2). It also supplies control solution to check that the meter is working properly, and software to download results from a computer.

URINE

> *I do not understand why it is that the glucose from the blood only spills into the urine above a certain level. I gather this level is known as the renal threshold – could you explain it for me in a little more detail?*

Urine is formed by filtration of blood in the kidneys. When the glucose concentration in the blood is below about 10 mmol/L, any glucose filtered into the urine is subsequently reabsorbed back into the bloodstream. When the level of glucose exceeds about 10 mmol/L (the renal threshold) more glucose is filtered than the body can reabsorb, and as a result it is passed in the urine. Once the level has exceeded 10 mmol/L, the amount of glucose in the urine will be proportional to the level of glucose in the blood. Below 10 mmol/L, however, there will be no glucose in the urine and, since the blood glucose level never exceeds 10 mmol/L in people without diabetes, they will not find glucose in the urine, unless they have a particular inherited condition called renal glycosuria.

What does it mean if I have a lot of ketones but no glucose on urine testing?

Testing for ketones in the urine can be rather confusing and, unless there are special reasons for doing it, we do not recommend it for routine use. Some people seem to develop ketones in the urine very readily, especially children, pregnant women and those who are dieting strictly to lose weight.

Usually if glucose and ketones appear together it indicates poor diabetes control, although this may pass off quickly so that glucose and ketones, present in the morning, may disappear by noon. If they are both a permanent feature, your diabetes needs to be better controlled, probably by increasing the insulin dose.

On rare occasions, ketones may appear in the urine without glucose. This is most likely to be found in the first morning specimen and probably occurs because the insulin taken the previous night is wearing off. Under these circumstances it is not serious and no action is needed.

Finally, ketones without glucose in the urine are very common in people who are trying to lose weight through calorie restriction. Anyone on a strict diet and losing weight will burn up body fat, which causes ketones to appear in the urine. Provided that there is no excess glucose in your urine, these ketones are of no concern and probably indicate that you are losing weight by breaking down body fat.

Why does one not always get a true blood glucose reading through a urine test (as in my case)?

In most people, urine contains glucose only when the glucose concentration in the blood is higher than a certain figure (usually 10 mmol/L), so below this level urine tests give no indication at all of the concentration of glucose in the blood. The level at which glucose spills out into the urine (the renal threshold, discussed earlier in this section) varies from one person to another and you can assess it in yourself only by making many simultaneous blood and urine glucose measurements. If you have a low renal threshold for glucose, you should abandon urine testing and rely entirely on blood tests to provide information about your diabetes. However, at early stages of Type 2 diabetes, when people are well controlled on diet alone, or perhaps with a single tablet, there may be a place for urine testing. Some people prefer this to pricking their finger for a blood glucose measurement and the strips have the advantage of being very much cheaper than blood glucose testing strips. If you use urine tests to monitor control of Type 2 diabetes, you should aim at keeping your urine free from glucose at all times and confirm with HbA_{1c} measurements that you are maintaining good control.

For some time now I have suffered from diabetes. I am curious to know what type of tests are made on my urine specimens when they are taken off to the laboratory.

Urine specimens are tested for several things but the most common are glucose, ketones and albumin (protein). These tests serve only as a spot check and are meant to complement your own tests performed at home. Clinics still tend to test the percentage of glucose in urine samples, even though the HbA_{1c} is a much better guide to diabetes control. The detection of ketones is of rather limited value since some people make ketones very easily and others almost not at all, but the presence of large amounts of ketones together with 2% glucose shows that the diabetes is very badly out of control.

The presence of protein in the urine can indicate either infection in the urine or the presence of some kidney disease, which in people with diabetes is likely to be diabetic nephropathy, a long-term complication (see Chapter 8). A more recent test is for microalbuminuria; the test detects microscopic amounts of albumin in the urine and can show signs of very early kidney damage.

I have a strong family history of diabetes. My daughter recently tested her urine and found 2% glucose. However, her blood glucose was only 8 mmol/L. She underwent a glucose tolerance test and this was normal. Could she have diabetes or could there be another reason why she is passing glucose in her water?

It is very unlikely that she has diabetes if a glucose tolerance test was normal. If she had glucose in her urine during the glucose tolerance test when all the blood glucose readings were strictly normal, then this would indicate that she has a low renal threshold for glucose (as discussed at the beginning of this section). If this is the correct diagnosis, it is important to find out whether she passes glucose in her urine first thing in the morning while fasting or only after she has eaten. People who pass glucose in their urine during the fasting state do not have an increased incidence of development of diabetes, and the condition (called renal glycosuria) is inherited. If, on the other hand, your daughter passes glucose in the urine only after meals containing starch and sugar, this condition sometimes progresses to diabetes.

HAEMOGLOBIN A$_{1C}$

When I last went to the clinic, I had a test for haemoglobin A$_{1c}$. What is this for and what are the normal values?

Haemoglobin A$_{1c}$ is a component of the red pigment of blood (haemoglobin A, or HbA) which carries oxygen from the lungs to the various organs in the body. The HbA$_{1c}$ is calculated as a percentage of total haemoglobin and can be measured by a variety of laboratory methods. HbA$_{1c}$ consists of HbA combined with glucose by a chemical link. The amount of HbA$_{1c}$ present is directly proportional to the average blood glucose during the 120-day life span of the HbA-containing red blood corpuscles in the circulating blood.

The test for HbA$_{1c}$ is the most successful so far developed to give an index of diabetes control. The blood glucose tests, which we have used for many years, fluctuate too erratically with injections, meals and other events for an isolated sample taken at one clinic visit to provide much information about overall control. HbA_{1c} averages out the peaks and troughs of the blood glucose over the previous two to three months.

Normal values vary a little from one laboratory to another and this can be a source of confusion as results from different clinics cannot be compared directly without the normal range known for each particular laboratory. (Diabetes UK is trying to correct this anomaly.) Normal values usually run between 4.5% and 6.1%, but you must check the normal range for your own laboratory. In someone with poorly controlled diabetes, or in whom diabetes is recently diagnosed, the value of HbA_{1c} may be as high as 15%, which reflects a consistently raised blood glucose over the preceding two to three months. If control is good, the HbA_{1c} will be in the target range of 6.5–7.5%, while someone who runs their blood glucose levels low by taking too much insulin may have a subnormal value, that is, below 6%. There is a move to change the way HbA_{1c} is reported from a percentage of haemoglobin to the new units called mmol/mol. The target range will be less than 48, which is the equivalent of less than 6.5%. To help with the change over, most laboratories will report the HbA_{1c} both as a percentage and in the new units.

I've just had a fructosamine test but I didn't like to ask what this was for. What is this test?

Fructosamine is the name of a test that is similar to HbA_{1c} in that it indicates the average level of glucose in the blood over a period of time, in this case the two to three weeks before the test is done (compared with the preceding two to three months for HbA_{1c}). It measures the amount of glucose linked to the proteins in the blood plasma (the straw-coloured fluid in which the red cells are suspended): the higher the blood glucose concentration, the higher will be the fructosamine. Its advantages are that it is usually quicker and cheaper for the laboratory to do. The normal values may vary from one laboratory to another depending on the way the analysis is performed; in general, a value of less than 300 micromol/litre is a typical laboratory's normal value. In order to make sure you don't get confused, we suggest that you pay particular attention to what is done in your clinic; please don't hesitate to ask and make quite sure you do know what is going on.

I have had diabetes for ten years and now take insulin. I have been attending the clinic regularly every three months and do regular blood glucose tests at home with my own meter. At my last clinic visit, the doctor I saw said that he did not need to see me again for a whole year because my HbA$_{1c}$ was consistently normal – why did he do this?

It sounds as though your doctor has great confidence in your ability to control your diabetes. As long as you can keep it this way, he clearly feels that seeing you once a year is sufficient. He can then spend more time with other people who are not as successful as you are. On the other hand, if you find the clinic visits helpful and motivating, it may be disappointing to be left 'on your own' for so long. You could see your practice nurse, who may be able to provide the support you need.

I am treated only by diet. I find it very difficult to stick to my diet or do the tests between the clinic visits but I am always very strict for the few days before I am seen at the clinic and my blood glucose test is usually normal. At my last clinic visit my blood glucose was 5 mmol/L but the doctor said he was very unhappy about my control because the HbA$_{1c}$ was too high at 10% – what did he mean?

Your experience demonstrates the usefulness of HbA$_{1c}$ testing, because you have been misleading yourself as well as your medical advisers about your ability to cope with your diabetes. The HbA$_{1c}$ has brought this to light. Because the HbA$_{1c}$ reflects your average blood glucose over the previous two to three months, your last-minute attempts to get your diabetes under control before your clinic visit were enough to bring the blood glucose down but the HbA_{1c} remained high.

My recent HbA_{1c} was said to be low at 6%. Blood glucose readings look all right, on average about 5 mmol/litre. The specialist asked me to set the alarm clock and check them at 3 a.m. – why is this?

A low HbA_{1c} suggests that at some stage your blood glucose levels are running unduly low. If you are not having hypoglycaemic attacks during the day, then it is possible that they are occurring at night and you are sleeping through them. By doing 3 a.m. blood glucose tests you should be able to determine whether this is so. Incidentally, you will only have to do these middle-of-the-night tests until you have established whether or not you are having hypos at night – they are not going to be a permanent part of your routine!

My diabetes is treated with diet and gliclazide tablets. By strict dieting I have lost weight down to slightly below my target figure. I am told that my HbA_{1c} test is still too high at 9% and does not seem to be falling despite the fact that I am still losing weight. I could not tolerate metformin and am very strict over what I eat. At the last clinic visit the doctor said that I am going to have to go onto insulin injections. I have been dreading this – is he right?

It is normal to dislike the idea of starting insulin injections but it sounds as if your diabetes is out of control and this is the reason for your weight loss. Since you cannot tolerate metformin, the only treatment available would be a glitazone. There is a 50% chance that this would bring your HbA_{1c} below the target of 7.5%. If this fails to help, the only option would be insulin. Naturally you are anxious about this but the chances are that you will find the injections easier than you fear. Most people do very well once they get used to the idea and feel much better once their blood sugars are lower.

DIABETES CLINICS

My GP is starting a diabetes clinic in the local group practice and tells me that I no longer need to attend the hospital clinic. It's much more convenient for me to go to see my GP but will this be all right?

You are fortunate that your general practitioner has a special interest in diabetes and has gone to the trouble of setting up a special clinic in the practice for this. Many GPs and practice nurses have had special training in diabetes and these general practice-based diabetes clinics are becoming more common. They usually work well as long as you have uncomplicated diabetes and are well controlled, but you should be aware of the sort of care you can expect: Diabetes UK's recommendations are given at the end of this section. We are sure that your hospital specialist will know about your GP's new clinic and may even attend it from time to time. If you have any anxieties, why not discuss them with your doctor?

My GP is keen to test my urine every year to 'look for evidence of kidney damage'. This sounds very frightening. Please explain.

The test goes by the name of microalbuminuria. For years nurses in diabetic clinics have asked for a urine sample which they test for protein. This is a crude test and is only positive when there is a lot of protein in the urine. The new test is very sensitive and detects minute traces of albumin (the body's most common protein). Research has shown that protein detected in such small amounts is the first sign of kidney damage but at this early stage it can be reversed. This damage can be slowed by keeping the blood pressure below 135/75 and controlling the blood glucose – HbA_{1c} 7% or less. The result of this test is often presented as a ratio of albumin (the protein) to creatinine, which corrects for the flow of urine at the time. The best result is to have a ratio of less than 0.5. The top limit of normal is usually quoted as 3.5 for women and 2.5 for men. If left untreated, the amount of protein in the urine will increase until it can be detected by conventional urine testing sticks. Over a period of years, this may progress to kidney failure and the possible need for dialysis or a kidney transplant. At the early stage of microalbuminuria, this process is reversible by control of blood pressure and glucose. There is good evidence that people with normal blood pressure and microalbuminuria can be protected by treatment with a tablet called an ACE inhibitor.

I have had diabetes for ten years and used to be seen in the hospital clinic once a year. Now my practice nurse has asked me to see her every three months. Is there an explanation?

When diabetes was regarded as a 'hospital condition', the clinics tended to be enormous and because of pressure of numbers, patients were normally seen every 6 or 12 months. It is universally agreed that everyone with diabetes should have an annual series of checks – known as the annual review – so the maximum time between appointments should be 12 months (see **What care to expect** in Figure 4.1). When the results of the UKPDS trial demonstrated the importance of good control in preventing complications, it became clear that regular contact with healthcare professionals was necessary to achieve and maintain tight control. Patients in these studies were seen every three months. Many primary care clinics have followed the UKPDS model and see patients every three to six months – or more frequently if there is a specific problem to be solved. It is important to have regular, structured diabetes care and the time between visits should be agreed between you and the doctor or nurse.

As a newly diagnosed person with diabetes what sort of care should I expect?

D iabetes UK issued a document in June 2000 called *What diabetes care to expect*. This has been updated recently but the basics haven't changed. The list should probably include a routine test for microalbuminuria – see the question above in this section. This document explains clearly what standards of care to expect and some of the guidelines from it are reproduced in Figure 4.1. If you would like a copy of the complete document, contact Diabetes UK (address in Appendix 2).

I have just heard that my appointment at the hospital diabetic clinic has been cancelled and that my GP will take over the care of my diabetes. Why is this?

O ver the last few years important changes have taken place in diabetes care. More patients are now treated in primary care, by GPs and practice nurses trained in the care of people with diabetes. Hospitals now concentrate on looking after more complex cases, including special circumstances such as pregnancy. In the past nearly all patients with diabetes were treated in hospital clinics but in the 1990s, as the number of people with Type 2 diabetes increased, there was a trend to encourage GPs and practice nurses to look after patients who did not need insulin. As they gained experience in diabetes, practice nurses began to start Type 2 patients on insulin and this has now become routine.

We are now more aware of the very strong link between Type 2 diabetes and heart disease and stroke. GPs are experienced at treating the risk factors for these conditions, namely high blood pressure and cholesterol, and are well placed to take overall responsibility for the care of patients with Type 2 diabetes. Those GPs and practice nurses who are confident with helping Type 2 patients adjust their insulin doses may take responsibility for some patients with Type 1 diabetes.

We welcome this trend to treat patients closer to home, with the obvious proviso that the system only works if GPs and practice nurses have the necessary training to look after people with diabetes and can call on specialists for support when they feel they need advice. Most surgeries now have a clinic for people with diabetes, run by a nurse or doctor with a special interest in treating this condition.

I have had diabetes for more than 20 years and throughout this time have been to the hospital diabetic clinic twice a year. I've now been told that I can no longer be seen at the hospital and that I must see my GP instead. As you can imagine, I am feeling rather anxious about this. What is the reason for the change?

We can understand your anxiety and will try to provide the reassurance you need, though of course that is difficult without knowing your local situation. The government is committed to altering the balance of diabetes care so that most of it is now carried out in GP surgeries. This has required additional education and many practice nurses and GPs have taken extra academic qualifications in diabetes. At the start of this process, GPs took on patients with Type 2 diabetes who were controlled by diet or tablets or both. Once they needed insulin, patients would be referred to the hospital clinic or diabetes specialist nurses, who would initiate insulin treatment. Such patients would often continue to come to the hospital indefinitely. The majority of health centres have now gained confidence and experience in the use of insulin and are happy to take on the care of their insulin-treated patients. Some people with complex medical problems will probably continue to be seen in hospital clinics.

Diabetes
UK

WHAT CARE TO EXPECT FROM YOUR HEALTHCARE TEAM

Whether you have just been diagnosed or had diabetes for some time it is important that you get regular high quality healthcare. This will help to ensure that your diabetes, blood pressure and blood fats are all kept in check as well as detecting any early signs of complications so that they can be caught and treated successfully.

To achieve the best possible diabetes care, you need to work together with healthcare professionals as equal members of your diabetes care team. It is essential that you understand your diabetes as well as possible so that you are an effective member of this team.

You need to discuss with your consultant or GP the roles and responsibilities of those providing your diabetes care and to identify the key members of your own diabetes care team.

MEMBERS OF YOUR HEALTHCARE TEAM

- yourself
- consultant physician/diabetologist
- GP
- practice nurse
- dietitian
- optometrist/ophthalmologist
- podiatrist/chiropodist
- psychologist
- other medical specialists
- pharmacist

You may see some members of your diabetes care team more often than others.

Figure 4.1

WHEN YOU HAVE JUST BEEN DIAGNOSED

When you have just been diagnosed, your diabetes care team should:

- Give you a full medical examination.
- Work with you to make a programme of care which suits you and includes diabetes management goals – this may take the form of a record for you to keep.
- Arrange for you to talk with a diabetes specialist nurse (or practice nurse) who will explain what diabetes is and discuss your individual treatment and the equipment you will need to use.
- Arrange for you to talk with a state registered dietitian, who will want to know what you usually eat, and will give you advice on how to fit your usual diet in with your diabetes – a follow-up meeting should be arranged for more detailed advice.
- Tell you about your diabetes and the beneficial effects of a healthy diet, exercise and good diabetes control.
- Discuss the effects of diabetes on your job, driving, insurance, prescription charges, and if you are a driver, whether you need to inform the DVLA and your insurance company.
- Provide you with regular and appropriate information and education, on food and footcare for example.
- Give you information about Diabetes UK services and details of your local Diabetes UK voluntary group.

WHEN YOUR DIABETES IS REASONABLY CONTROLLED

Once your diabetes is reasonably controlled, you should:

- Have access to your diabetes care team at least once a year – in this session, take the opportunity to discuss how your diabetes affects you as well as your diabetes control.
- Be able to contact any member of your diabetes care team for specialist advice, in person or by phone.
- Have further education sessions when you are ready for them.
- Have a formal medical annual review once a year with a doctor experienced in diabetes.

Figure 4.1 (*continued*)

ON A REGULAR BASIS

On a regular basis, your diabetes care team should:

- Provide continuity of care, ideally from the same doctors and nurses – if this is not possible , the doctors or nurses who you are seeing should be fully aware of your medical history and background.
- Work with you to continually review your care programme, including your diabetes management goals.
- Let you share in decisions about your treatment or care.
- Let you manage your own diabetes in hospital after discussion with your doctor, if you are well enough to do so and that is what you wish.
- Organise pre- and post-pregnancy advice, together with an obstetric hospital team, if you are planning to become, or already are, pregnant.
- Encourage a carer to visit with you, to keep them up to date on diabetes so that they can make informed judgements about diabetes care.
- Encourage the support of friends, partners and/or relatives.
- Provide you with education sessions and appointments if you wish.
- Give you advice on the effects of diabetes and its treatments when you are ill or taking other medication.

WITH YOUR TREATMENT

If you are treated by insulin injections you should:

- Have frequent visits showing how to inject, look after your insulin and syringes and dispose of sharps (needles). You should also be shown how to test your blood glucose and test for ketones and be informed what the results mean and what to do about them.
- Be given supplies of, or a prescription for the medication and equipment you need.
- Discuss hypoglycaemia (hypos): when and why they may happen and how to deal with them.

Figure 4.1 (*continued*)

If you are treated by tablets you should:

- Be given instruction on blood or urine testing and have explained what the results mean and what to do about them.
- Be given supplies of, or a prescription for the medication and equipment you need.
- Discuss hypoglycaemia (hypos): when and why they may happen and how to deal with them.

If you are treated by diet alone you should:

- Be given instruction on blood or urine testing and have explained what the results mean and what to do about them.
- Be given supplies of equipment you may need.

Figure 4.1 (*continued*)

I've heard a lot of talk about the Diabetes NSF. What is it and how will it affect me?

Several years ago the Department of Health set up a scheme called the National Service Framework (NSF), which set out standards of care for a number of long-term conditions, such as heart disease and mental health. Diabetes was chosen as an important condition for which clear standards of care were needed.

The first section of the Diabetes NSF was published in 2001. This contained the agreed Standards of Care and was followed by the Delivery Strategy, which was published in 2003. This was designed to be implemented over several years with all targets achieved by 2013. The first target to be met was screening for retinopathy by digital photography to be available for all people with diabetes by the end of 2007.

The NSF Standards are printed in this chapter. The Delivery Strategy is a 40-page document which lacks a summary. However, it contains some worthy aspirations and we hope there will be funding to make these a reality. The NSF website: www.dh.gov.uk/PolicyAndGuidance/HealthAndSocialCareTopics/Diabetes has the document.

The key elements proposed in this *Delivery Strategy* are:

- setting up a local diabetes network, or similar robust mechanism, which involves identifying local leaders and appointing and resourcing network managers, clinical champions and a person(s) with diabetes to champion the views of local people

- reviewing the local baseline assessment, establishing and promulgating local implementation arrangements with a trajectory to reach the standards

- participating in comparative local and national audit

- undertaking a local workforce skills profile of staff involved in the care of people with diabetes and developing education and training programmes with the local Workforce Development Confederation.

It also reflects targets in *Improvement, Expansion and Reform: the next three years*:

- ensuring a systematic eye-screening programme to national standards

- putting in place registers, education and advice, to support systematic treatment regimens.

The *Delivery Strategy* offers a framework for the NHS to build capacity to:

- put in place building blocks for the NHS to reach the National Service Framework (NSF) standards over the next ten years

- deliver the national targets.

I've been told my GP will be paid extra if my HbA$_{1c}$ is less that 7.5%. Can this be true?

This may sound a bit surprising, but it is true that the government has recently changed the way GPs are paid by negotiating a new contract based partly on the level of care achieved. For many conditions there is evidence that if certain targets are reached, the outcome for patients is greatly improved. Thus, we know that for people with diabetes the risk of complications is significantly reduced if the HbA$_{1c}$ is less than 7.5%. Similarly, a blood pressure of less than 140/80 and a cholesterol of less than 4 mmol/L will reduce the risk of heart attack and stroke. The government believes that providing GPs with incentives to achieve these targets will drive up standards of care. The early signs are that this strategy has had some success.

My GP and practice nurse are putting pressure on me to improve control of my diabetes. I have heard that this is because they will be paid more if I get my HbA$_{1c}$ down to 7.4%. Why should I do this just to increase my doctor's income?

Although you may feel that lowering your HbA$_{1c}$ is more for your doctor's benefit than yours, it is important to remember that the reason the government introduced these targets for GPs is that there is strong evidence to show that people with diabetes have fewer health problems if their HbA$_{1c}$ is less than 7.5%. Thus, it is in your own interests to improve the control of your diabetes. It is sad that the targets, introduced as a way of improving care for people with diabetes, have altered the doctor–patient relationship and given some people the impression that their doctor is more concerned about income than patient care.

BLOOD GLUCOSE SELF-MONITORING GUIDELINES

These guidelines were developed by Coventry PCT

Education and lifestyle interventions	• Advice on diet, exercise and smoking habit key interventions at diagnosis and beyond • If necessary, patients should receive education relevant to **appropriate** testing, **understanding when** to test and **what** to do with the result	ALL PATIENTS WHO ARE SELF-MONITORING SHOULD BE ENCOURAGED TO USE THE MINIMUM NUMBER OF TESTS REQUIRED TO KEEP CONTROL	
Newly diagnosed Type 2 patient + **diet control only** Recommended regime: **A**	• Self-monitoring may be required at diagnosis or as necessary depending on overall diabetic control and management plan • Self-monitoring may **not be necessary** if control is acceptable (e.g. HbA$_{1c}$ to target) • Healthcare professional should advise patient when self-monitoring becomes necessary	Urine testing may be appropriate for some patients in this group provided HbA$_{1c}$ targets are achieved	Typical weekly strip usage **0–6**

Figure 4.2

Type 2 patient, prescribed oral therapy Recommended regimes: ## A, B, C	• Re-assess patient need and educate prior to initiation of single oral therapy or combined treatment • If self-monitoring is necessary, the healthcare professional should tailor monitoring regime to individual patient need, depending on diabetic control • Special focus on testing to prevent hypoglycaemia, especially in sulphonylurea therapy	If starting self-monitoring at this stage teach patient before initiating new therapy	Typical weekly strip usage ## 0–6
Type 2 patient, prescribed insulin Recommended regimes: ## B, D, E	• Self-monitoring is recommended in all cases with daily testing on initiation of insulin • Once a patient is stable, frequency of profiles can be reduced to 1–2 days a week or daily at varying times (week profile)	Stable patients are those whose blood glucose varies little from day to day and who are not having intensive changes of treatment	Typical weekly strip usage ## 4–28
Type 1 patients Recommended regimes ## E, F	• Self-monitoring is strongly recommended in all cases • Self-monitoring should be used to adjust insulin dose before meals where this is appropriate (e.g. basal bolus regime, pump therapy) • Self-monitoring in Type 1 diabetes may only be required on 1–2 days per week in stable patients and depending on patient's daily routine		Typical weekly strip usage ## 8–28

Figure 4.2 (*continued*)

Examples of typical self-monitoring regimes

Regime A	One or two tests a week
Regime B	Once daily at various times (week profile)
Regime C	Two tests daily
Regime D	Four tests at different times on one day (day profile)
Regime E	Day profile twice a week
Regime F	Test before meals and at bedtime each day

- Urine testing is appropriate in those:
    - where blood glucose monitoring is not possible
    - or the patient has a preference not to blood test
- HbA$_{1c}$ target = below 7.5%
- Increase testing frequency during:
    - pregnancy
    - times of illness
    - changes in therapy
    - changes in routine
    - times of poor control
    - when at risk of hypoglycaemia
    - also to rule out hypoglycaemia, especially when driving.

Blood glucose monitoring targets

Fasting	4–6 mmol/L	Bedtime	5–10 mmol/L
Pre-prandial	4–6 mmol/L	Post-prandial	<10 mmol/L

- Self-monitoring does not replace regular HbA$_{1c}$ testing , which remains the gold standard test, and should only be used in conjunction with appropriate therapy as part of integrated care.

Figure 4.2 (*continued*)

5 | Life with diabetes

This chapter attempts to answer all the questions about issues that affect daily living when you have diabetes. It covers a broad sweep ranging from sport and holidays to surgical operations and illness. The section *Other illnesses* should be read early on, so that you will know how to react if you are struck down by a bad attack of flu. All car drivers should read the section *Driving*. At the end of the chapter is a miscellaneous section on issues which did not fall into the main sections: questions on electrolysis, ear piercing and identity bracelets for example. After reading this chapter, you will realise that there are very few activities that are barred to people with diabetes. Provided that you understand the condition, you should be able to do almost anything you wish.

SPORTS

I used to enjoy swimming, but have been worried about going back to the pool since I have been on insulin. What if I had a hypo?

A hypo while swimming can be serious and you are right to be concerned about it. However, don't let your concern stop you swimming. There are certain simple rules that all people taking insulin should follow before swimming; these will allow you to swim with complete safety.

- Never swim alone.

- Tell your companions to pull you out of the water if you behave oddly or are in difficulty.

- Keep glucose tablets or Lucozade on the side of the pool.

- Get out of the water immediately at the first signs of a hypo.

If you are a keen swimmer and want to take up scuba diving, the British Sub-Aqua Club does impose some restrictions. It requires people taking insulin who wish to scuba dive to have an annual medical review, to be free of any long-term complications of diabetes, and insists that they always dive with another person who does not have diabetes. You can contact the Club for more details – the address is in Appendix 2.

Can I take part in all or any forms of sport?

The vast majority of sports are perfectly safe for people with diabetes. The problem lies in those sports where loss of control due to a hypo could be dangerous, not only to you but to fellow participants or spectators. Swimming is an example of a potentially dangerous sport but, if you take certain precautions it is safe (see previous question). However, in some sports (such as motor racing) the risk of serious injury in the case of a hypo is even greater. The governing bodies of such high-risk sports discourage people with diabetes from taking part. Discouragement does not necessarily mean a total ban – the restrictions may vary depending on whether you are on diet, diet and tablets, or insulin. You can always contact the appropriate governing body to ask what (if any) restrictions they impose. Skiing is discussed in the section on *Holidays and travel* later in this chapter.

Are people with diabetes allowed to go parachuting? I want to do a sponsored parachute jump to raise money for charity.

You can probably do your sponsored jump, but it will depend on your current treatment. If you are on diet alone, or on diet and biguanides, restrictions are minimal. If you are on sulphonylureas or insulin the restrictions are much greater – you will need a medical certificate to state that you are well controlled, and you will be permitted to jump only in tandem. The British Parachute Association (address in Appendix 2) can give you more information about this.

As a 30-year-old with diabetes, can I join a keep fit class or do a work-out at home?

Keeping fit is important for everybody. Like everyone else, if you are unused to exercise, you should build up the exercises slowly week by week to avoid damaging muscles or tendons. Remember that exercise usually has the effect of lowering blood glucose, so you may need to reduce the insulin dose or take extra carbohydrate beforehand (see the first question in this section).

I have Type 2 diabetes and am overweight and not well controlled despite a maximum dose of tablets. I have been advised to join an exercise class. Will this be worth the effort?

It has been shown beyond doubt that, if you can change your lifestyle and improve your fitness by taking regular exercise, this will have a major beneficial effect on the control of your diabetes and your risk of heart disease.

I take insulin and jog quite a bit. I would like to try running a marathon. Have you any advice on the subject?

It is perfectly possible to run a marathon while taking insulin for diabetes. We suggest that you progress gradually from jogging short distances to a full marathon distance. Everyone is different and you will need to discover by trial and error how your body responds to endurance exercise. It may not sound very easy but you will have to check your blood glucose levels frequently to find out how to match your energy intake and expenditure. You will need plenty of 'slow' carbohydrate (e.g. porridge) to maintain your energy levels. Since endurance exercise increases insulin sensitivity, you will probably find that you need to take much less insulin while running long distances. You should carry glucose in the form of tablets or high-energy glucose drinks.

Diabetes UK produces factsheets on long-distance running and some other sports. Once you have reached the required standard, you should think of joining Diabetes UK's team for the London Marathon.

EATING OUT

My wife and I entertain a great deal and we often go out for meals in a restaurant. I have recently been started on insulin for diabetes. How am I going to cope with eating out?

Nowadays people with diabetes usually eat similar food to anyone who is following a healthy lifestyle. Although you should normally try to avoid foods that are obviously high in sugar and fat, this may be difficult when you are visiting friends.

Restaurants or takeaways should pose less of a problem as you can select suitable dishes from the menu. Many people using a basal bolus regimen choose to take extra short-acting insulin to cover the extra food they are eating. Estimating the amount of carbohydrate in the food and deciding how much insulin you need is a skill which develops with experience. In an earlier section (see p. 25) we have talked about the DAFNE method, which teaches you how to calculate your insulin dose accurately. If you are uncertain about the size of portion you will be given in a restaurant you should wait until you see what is on your plate before deciding on the dose of insulin.

Sometimes people worry about how they are going to give their injections when they are away from home. With an insulin pen there should be no difficulty and most people are able to give the insulin discreetly at the table when the food arrives. Do not take your evening dose of insulin before leaving home in case the meal is delayed.

FASTING AND DIABETES

As a Muslim I wish to fast during Ramadan. Is this possible?

People with diabetes who fast during Ramadan may experience large swings in blood glucose levels, as a result of the long gaps between meals and the consumption of large quantities of carbohydrate-rich foods during the non-fasting hours. Therefore, if you have diabetes, you may be exempt from fasting. However, many people with diabetes do not want to be exempted from a religious observance that they feel strongly about. If you have Type 2 diabetes and are treated by diet alone there should be no problem with fasting during Ramadan. However, there will be major changes in the pattern of eating during this month, which may affect your diabetes. If you are treated with insulin injections, sulphonylurea tablets, or a combination of the two, you should discuss how fasting may affect your blood glucose control with your diabetes team, before Ramadan begins.

If you are on sulphonylurea tablets and are fasting during Ramadan, you can take the tablet at the end of the fast, within 30 minutes of starting your evening meal. You must not miss the sehti, the meal before sunrise, if you are to avoid hypoglycaemia later in the day. Repaglinide (NovoNorm®) can be particularly useful, as it need only be taken with a meal, thus requiring no change of treatment during Ramadan.

HOLIDAYS AND TRAVEL

Do you have any simple rules for people with diabetes going abroad for holidays?

Here is a checklist of things to take with you.
- Insulin (or tablets)
- Syringes or insulin pen and needles
- Test strips (and finger pricker) and/or meter
- Identification bracelet/necklace/card
- Glucose tablets
- Starchy carbohydrate in case meals are delayed
- Glucagon

- Medical insurance

- European Health Insurance Card (EHIC), which has replaced Form E111, if travelling inside the EU (see question on p. 157)

- Glucogel (Hypostop).

Is it safe for someone with diabetes to take travel sickness tablets?

Travel sickness pills do not upset diabetes, although they may make you sleepy so be careful if you are driving. On the other hand, vomiting can upset diabetes so it is worthwhile trying to avoid travel sickness. If you do become sick, the usual rules apply. Continue to take your normal dose of insulin and take carbohydrate in some palatable liquid form, such as a sugary drink. Test your blood glucose regularly.

We are going on holiday and wish to take a supply of insulin and glucagon with us. How should I store them both for the journey and in the hotel?

Insulin is very stable and will keep for one month at room temperature in our temperate climate. However, it does not like extremes of temperature and can be damaged if kept too long at high temperatures or if frozen. It is best to carry your supplies in more than one piece of luggage in case one suitcase goes astray.

In these days of increased airport security, people traveling with normal equipment needed to manage their diabetes are being challenged for evidence that their materials are bona fide, which can be extremely irritating. Security staff need to see a list on official (hospital or practice) headed notepaper of the items to be carried. Alternatively you can obtain an insulin user's identification card online or by phone from Diabetes UK at a cost of £5. Also available from Diabetes UK is a treatment identity card for £1.50.

If you are travelling by air you should keep your insulin in your hand luggage – temperatures in the luggage hold of an aircraft usually fall below freezing and insulin left in luggage there could be damaged. Insulin manufacturers say it is stable for one month at 25°C (77°F), so it is perfectly safe to keep insulin with your luggage on the average holiday. Avoid the glove compartment or the boot of your car where very high temperatures can be reached. In tropical conditions your stock of insulin should be kept in the fridge.

Storage of glucagon is no problem as this comes as a powder with a vial of water for dilution. It is very stable and can survive extremes of heat and cold.

I am travelling to the Middle East on business and have diabetes, which is well controlled on tablets. Can you give me any tips about diabetes and travel?

There should not be any particular worries about travelling abroad. There is the obvious advice about taking adequate supplies of all your tablets and testing equipment. Sometimes airport security can be a bit wary of blood testing kits, though it is hard to imagine how anyone could perpetrate a scare with a finger pricker. It would probably be worth asking your GP for a letter on headed paper to certify the need for this equipment. Alternatively for a modest fee, Diabetes UK will provide you with a treatment identity card.

The greatest problem concerning business travel and diabetes is the difficulty in obtaining normal food in high-grade hotels. The goal of hotel chefs seems to be to tempt everyone to eat twice as much high-calorie food, preferably containing plenty of unsuitable fats, as they need. Try to seek out items on the menu which are (relatively) healthy. Remember, you don't have to finish every plateful – especially in countries where excessive portions are the norm.

I would like to go on a skiing holiday. Is it safe for me to ski, skate and toboggan? Should I take special precautions?

It is as safe for someone with diabetes to ski and enjoy other winter sports as it is for anyone else. Accidents do occur and it is essential to take out adequate insurance to cover all medical expenses. Read the small print in the insurance form carefully to ensure that it does not exclude pre-existing conditions like diabetes, or require them to be declared. In this case you should contact the insurance company and if necessary take out extra medical cover for your diabetes. Diabetes UK can provide travel insurance that will cover your diabetes (see Appendix 2). Physical activity increases the likelihood of hypos so always carry glucose and a snack as you may be delayed, especially if you are injured. Never go without a sensible companion who knows you have diabetes and understands what to do if you have a hypo.

Do make sure your ski boots are properly fitted, particularly if you have any degree of neuropathy. Poorly fitting boots are a very common cause of foot damage and ulceration.

Is sunbathing all right for people with diabetes?

Of course people with diabetes can sunbathe. Lying around doing nothing may put your blood glucose up a little, especially if you overeat as most people do on holiday. So keep up your usual tests as you may need extra insulin. On the other hand, increasing the temperature of the skin may speed up the absorption of the insulin and can lead to hypos, so be prepared for changes. Remember that sunbathing can increase the risk of skin cancer whether or not you have diabetes, so always take sensible precautions to avoid sunburn by covering up, in the middle of the day particularly, and using sunscreen with a high protection factor.

As I have diabetes should I be vaccinated when going abroad?

People with diabetes should have exactly the same vaccinations as anyone else. You are no more or less likely to contract illnesses abroad but, if you do become ill, the consequences could be more serious. In addition to the necessary vaccinations, it is very important to take protective tablets against malaria if you are going to a tropical area where this disease is found. More cases of this potentially serious disease are being seen in this country, usually in travellers recently returned from Africa or the Far East.

I am going to work in the Middle East for six months. What can I do if my insulin is not available in the country where I am working?

If you are working abroad for six months only, it should be quite easy to take enough insulin to last you this length of time. Stored in an ordinary fridge it should keep – but make sure that you are not supplied with insulin near the end of its shelf life. The expiry date is printed on each box of insulin.

Most types of insulin are available in the Middle East, but you may have to make do with a different brand name or even insulin from a different source (pig, cow or human). Understandably, porcine insulin may be hard to obtain in strict Muslim countries. U100 insulin may be difficult to obtain outside the UK, USA, Australia, New Zealand, South Africa and parts of the Far East. Many European countries stock insulin in 40 units/mL only and special syringes for use with U40 insulin will have to be obtained. Diabetes UK can tell you which strength insulin is used in each country.

*My husband has just been offered an excellent post in Uruguay,
which he would love to accept. He is worried about my diabetes
there and especially about the availability of my insulin.
Can you let me know if my insulin can be sent by post?*

It should be possible to obtain an equivalent type of insulin to
your own in most parts of the world. If you are keen to keep up
your normal supplies, Hypoguard Ltd will despatch syringes and
equipment for testing blood and urine to all parts of the world.
Unfortunately Hypoguard is not able to handle insulin. You might
be able to make arrangements with a high street chemist who would
be prepared to send insulin by post. John Bell & Croyden in London
will send insulin abroad. The address is in Appendix 2.

*My friends and I are going to Spain to work next year.
Can you tell me what I should take with me and whether
I would have to pay if I needed to see a doctor?*

It is now common for people from the UK to live in other European
countries for long periods, if not for good. Generally speaking,
professional diabetes care is excellent in the fully developed countries
and you should expect the same process of screening for complications and help with diabetes as in the UK. Before you go abroad, you
should ask your doctor for a full report of your medical condition.
This should include the following:

- Details of insulin and method of injecting (e.g. type of penfill);
- Name of blood glucose testing strips;
- Recent blood pressure measurement;
- All other medication – using official rather than brand names,
  e.g. rosiglitazone rather than Avandia;
- Results of recent blood tests (HbA$_{1c}$, creatinine, cholesterol);
- Microalbuminuria test result;

- Latest retinal screening result – if any abnormalities, try to obtain a digital record of the photographs by email or on CD;
- Results of latest foot screening;
- Details of any known complications of diabetes.

Before you go abroad prepare well: take spares of insulin pens, testing equipment and so on, and keep spares separate from the main supply in case your luggage is lost.

Medical attention is free in all European Union countries, although you should obtain a European Health Insurance Card (EHIC) which replaces the old E111 certificate. You can order an EHIC online for £15. For longer stays abroad, you should contact the DSS. For countries outside the EU, you should insure your health before you go. Diabetes UK Careline can help you with this (see Chapter 10 for contact details).

I take insulin and need to fly to the USA. How do I cope with the changing time zones?

The most important advice when travelling long distance is to test your blood glucose more frequently than usual – at least every four to five hours. This may be inconvenient but travel is often unpredictable and curious things happen to diabetes control. The only way to keep safe is to test often, even if you're not normally a frequent tester. If you do have a bad hypo while aboard, the cabin crew will have to deal with it and they may not be particularly knowledgeable about diabetes.

If you take basal bolus insulin (short-acting insulin with each meal and long-acting insulin at bedtime) you should continue to take short-acting insulin each time you eat. If you take background (basal) insulin in two divided doses, it should be simple to swap round the morning and evening doses in the new time zone. However, if you only have a single daily injection of background insulin at bedtime, you need to decide whether or not to change the time you have this injection. If it is a short trip, you should continue to have background insulin at the same UK time as normal. However, if you are spending more than a week in the new time zone, it would be worth moving the time of the injection to bedtime. For instance, the East coast of USA is five hours behind UK time and you are likely to arrive in the afternoon, though your body clock will think it is five hours later. Provided you have short-acting insulin every four hours, you should be able to delay your background insulin till bedtime. If you are travelling in the opposite direction, the interval between long-acting injections will be shorter than usual so you may need to reduce the first dose of background insulin on arrival. If you underestimate the amount of insulin you need you can always correct with a small dose of short-acting insulin later. The key to the problem is frequent testing.

I am on twice-daily mixtures of insulin and am flying to Los Angeles on holiday. How will the change in time affect my diabetes?

If your diabetes is not well controlled on your present insulin, this could be an opportunity to change to a more flexible insulin regime. However, if you are well controlled on premixed insulin, there are ways of adjusting your insulin to the conditions. It would be sensible to ask your GP for a supply of short-acting insulin (Humalog® or NovoRapid®) which you can take if your blood sugars start to rise. Mixed insulin, which is mainly long-acting insulin, is not effective at reducing the blood glucose rapidly. The advice about blood testing (see previous question) applies and if at any time your glucose rises above 12 mmol/litre you should take insulin every four hours, preferably before a meal. The dose will depend on how much insulin you normally take in a day. Once you have arrived, continue to take short-acting insulin every four to six hours until you reach a time when you would normally take your premixed insulin – usually breakfast and evening meal. You can then go back to your normal insulin doses, though you must continue to test frequently as holidays are notorious for upsetting control of blood glucose. For specific advice, you should speak to your GP or diabetes specialist nurse.

TRAVEL TIPS

Flying across time zones can be confusing for anyone, and makes it difficult to know which meal you are eating. When travelling keep to the following rules.

- Do not aim at perfect control. You have to be flexible especially on international flights. A hypo while travelling can be very inconvenient.

- Be prepared to check your blood glucose if you are at all worried and unsure how much insulin you need.

- In general, airlines are prepared to make special allowances for people with diabetes and cabin crew will do their best to help. Airlines say that they like to be warned in advance.

- Most experienced travellers avoid special 'diabetic' meals which are usually very low in carbohydrate.

- Take two watches and keep one on UK time while you make the change in injection times. This will help you work out when you would be taking your insulin at home and you can then make gradual changes in injection times until you are synchronised with your new time zone.

Figure 5.1

WORK

Can I take a job involving shift work?

Many people combine shift work with good control of their blood glucose. Shift work does, however, demand a little extra care as most insulin regimens are designed round a 24-hour day. Shift workers usually complain that they are just settling into one routine when everything changes and they have to start again. It is hard to generalise about shift work as there are so many different patterns but, if you follow these rules, things should work out all right.

- Aim at an injection of short- and intermediate-acting insulin every 12–16 hours, or use a basal bolus regimen. This way of giving insulin makes it much simpler to plan for shift work.

- Try to eat a good meal after each injection.

- If there is a gap of six to eight hours when you are changing from one shift to another, take some short-acting insulin followed by a meal.

- Because your pattern of insulin and food is constantly changing, you will have to do more blood glucose measurements than normal, as you cannot assume that one day is very much like another.

- If your blood glucose results are not good, be prepared to make changes in your dose of insulin. You will soon become an expert about your own diabetes.

How can I cope with my diabetes if I work irregular hours as a sales rep?

Just as in shift work, many people manage to combine an irregular work pattern with good diabetes control. Those who lead an erratic lifestyle usually find that the basal bolus regimen gives them more freedom as it will allow them to miss or delay a meal without risk of a hypo. The basal bolus regimen is much easier to deliver using an insulin pen (see section *Insulin pens* in Chapter 3).

If you take twice-daily insulin and have a normal blood glucose before lunch, you are likely to go hypo unless you eat at the right time. You will not be able to afford the luxury of missing meals completely but it is always possible to have a few biscuits or even a sweet drink if you are getting past your normal eating time.

The occupational hazard of all sales reps, with diabetes or otherwise, is the mileage that they clock up each year on the roads. With modern blood glucose meters, it should be possible to avoid the dangers of hypoglycaemia while driving.

The rules for driving are:

- Always check your blood glucose before driving;

- If it is low, eat or take a glucose drink before you drive;

- Always carry food in your car and have some immediately if you feel warning of a hypo;

- If you think you may be hypo, pull off the road immediately, stop the car, turn off the ignition and remove the key;

- Do not resume driving until you are sure your blood glucose is in the normal range.

Should I warn fellow employees that I might be subject to hypos?

It is never easy to give personal information to workmates, but unfortunately hypos do happen at work, especially when a person first starts using insulin. You should warn your workmates that, if they find you acting in a peculiar way, they must persuade you to take some sugar. Warn them also that you may not be very cooperative at the time and may even resist their attempts to help. It is difficult to admit to colleagues that you have diabetes but, if you keep it a secret, you run the risk of causing a scare by having a bad hypo.

The natural response of your workmates will be to dial 999 and you may be taken to hospital by ambulance for treatment. You can probably avoid this worst-case scenario by giving your colleagues some useful diabetes education.

My husband's hours of work can be very erratic. Sometimes he only gets three or four hours' sleep instead of his normal eight hours. Can you tell me what effect lack of sleep has on diabetes?

Lack of sleep in itself will not affect diabetes although, if your husband is under great pressure, his blood glucose may be either higher or lower than usual. The real problem with working under a strain is the tendency to ignore diabetes completely and assume that it will look after itself. Unfortunately a few minutes of each day have to be spent checking blood glucose, eating a snack or giving insulin. These minutes are well spent.

I developed diabetes five months ago, one week after I had started a new job. I am coming to the end of my six-month probation period and have been given two weeks' notice because they say I cannot do shift work when I have diabetes. Can you help?

This is a sad story and a good example of ignorant prejudice against people with diabetes. Of course there are many people on shift work who maintain good control – although it does require a bit of extra thought. You may well have a case under the Disability Discrimination Act and you should seek advice from your local Citizen's Advice Bureau. If you are using the basal bolus insulin regime, there is no reason why you should not be able to adjust your insulin to your shifts. It may take a bit of juggling, but many people taking insulin manage in this way without any problem.

*I am a pub manager and have had diabetes for the past 19
years but my employers are now making me redundant.
Apparently, their insurers cannot accept me for a permanent
position owing to my diabetes. Who can help strengthen my
case?*

We know of several publicans with diabetes who successfully run pubs and still keep their diabetes under good control. However, people who work in licensed premises are at greater risk of drinking more alcohol than average, and heavy drinkers are in danger from hypos (see the section *Alcohol* later in this chapter). We wonder if you have been having frequent hypos, which has made it difficult to continue in your present occupation. Ask your doctor and Diabetes UK to lobby on your behalf and seek legal advice from your local Citizen's Advice Bureau.

*I have been refused a job with a large company because of
my diabetes. Have I sufficient grounds to take proceedings
against them for discrimination?*

The Disability Discrimination Act covers people with diabetes but taking a company to court can be difficult. Unfortunately this sort of discrimination does happen, especially in large organisations, although it can be very difficult to prove. The support of your own diabetes team will be important if you wish to take proceedings under the Disability Discrimination Act.

Diabetes UK has had discussions with medical officers responsible for occupational health in several large organisations. There is useful information on the Diabetes UK website, though it dates back to 2001.

OTHER ILLNESSES

I have recently had a severe cough and cold and have been given 'diabetic' cough medicine by the doctor. Since then my blood glucose has been very high. Could this be due to the medicine?

Antibiotic syrup and cough linctus are often blamed for making diabetes worse during an illness such as flu or a chest infection. In fact a dose of antibiotic syrup only contains about 5 g of sugar and will have very little effect on your blood glucose. It is the illness itself that unbalances the diabetes. In general, medication from your doctor will not upset your diabetes.

Any infection or serious illness will cause a rise in blood glucose and it is important to test your blood if you feel unwell. If you are taking insulin you will probably need to increase the dose during the illness and it is very important to continue regular insulin injections *even if you are not eating.* If you are vomiting and unable to keep fluids down you will need hospital admission for intravenous fluids. Vomiting can sometimes be a sign of ketoacidosis, which may be fatal if untreated.

The rules for illness are:

- Test blood at least four times a day;

- If tests are high take extra doses of short-acting insulin;

- If the tests are low, take a sugary drink such as Lucozade to treat the hypo;

- Never stop insulin.

It is of course possible to get over a bad cold by carrying on with your normal dose of insulin and accepting bad control for a few days. However, this means that your mouth and nose will be slightly dehydrated and it may take longer before you feel back to normal. You will probably feel better more quickly if you adjust your insulin and try to keep the blood glucose near normal.

I have noticed that I suffer from more colds since developing diabetes. Could this be due to the diabetes?

Many people make this observation, but there is no real reason why the common cold should be more common in diabetes. However, a relatively minor cold may upset your diabetes control and lead to several extra days of feeling unwell (see previous question). This may make it a more memorable event. To repeat the previous advice, never stop insulin.

What is the best treatment for someone suffering from hay fever? I understand that some products can cause drowsiness, which could affect my balance and be confused with a hypo.

You can use exactly the same treatment for your hay fever as people without diabetes, as it does not affect your control. Antihistamines are often used for hay fever and these may make you feel sleepy, but this should be easy to distinguish from a hypo. Remember that, if you are on antihistamines, you should be very cautious about drinking alcohol. Hay fever can also be alleviated by using a nasal spray to reduce the sensitivity of the membranes in the nose.

I have just been in hospital with anaphylactic shock from a bee sting. I have diabetes controlled with tablets and wondered if this had anything to do with the severity of my reaction?

There is no connection between diabetes and allergy to bees.

My husband is on tablets for diabetes and normally has good control. He is prone to chest infections and these seem to upset his blood sugars. What should he do?

This can be a really difficult problem. Of course if your husband is ill enough to need hospital admission, he should be given insulin while his sugars are running high. At home, this is not as simple because there is no way of knowing what dose of insulin he may require, and an inadequate dose of insulin may even make matters worse. In a perfect world he would have insulin for the duration of his illness but in reality it is acceptable for him to run high sugars for a day or so, in the expectation that they will soon settle down spontaneously. In a longer-lasting illness, he will need insulin if the sugars are consistently high and there will be time to adjust the insulin dose in response to the blood glucose measurements.

Chest infections and asthma are often treated with steroids, which can cause a major rise in the blood glucose; see question on medications on p. 179.

Since I was told I have Type 2 diabetes, I have been very depressed. Is there any link between depression and diabetes?

People vary greatly in their response to learning that they have diabetes; some are able to adjust to their new condition easily, while others find it hard to accept. We wonder what input you have received from your doctor or nurse to help you cope with this unpleasant news. We often hear of people who are told they have diabetes in a matter-of-fact way, and then see the practice nurse who gives them basic information about diabetes, sometimes backed up with some reading material. However, they leave the session feeling that their own fears and concerns have not been addressed. Such people often become angry and get the impression they have been responsible for their own diabetes. These negative emotions often cause depression and a belief that they can do nothing to improve the situation.

We support the DESMOND approach (see p. 27) where a group of people recently diagnosed with diabetes meet with an educator who is trained to listen as well as to teach. In the opening session, people are invited to tell their own story and this leads to a feeling of solidarity within the group. After learning basic facts about food and diabetes, including the effect this may have on their future health, members of the group are encouraged to set their own goals for improving their health. When first diagnosed with diabetes, it is often difficult to work out whether the condition is serious or trivial. The DESMOND process helps people get diabetes into perspective and allows them to make informed lifestyle choices regarding food and exercise. It also provides the reassurance of meeting other people with diabetes, who are living through the same difficult experience. Other centres have developed education programmes along similar lines to DESMOND.

I have heard that people with diabetes are more likely to be depressed. Is this true?

This sounds like a simple question but it is not easy to answer. Many research studies have shown that the majority of people with diabetes have a normal quality of life, unless they are affected by complications which interfere with daily living. You would probably predict that a lifelong disease, which puts extra demands on people, would lead to depression but it is hard to prove that this is actually the case.

On the other hand, there are many people who already have a serious psychological disease such as depression, anxiety or an eating disorder, who then develop diabetes. Whatever the cause of their depression, people who feel negative about themselves cannot summon up the energy required to look after their diabetes and it is more difficult for them to achieve good control.

How does stress and worry affect diabetes? I spend many hours studying and find that, if I study too long, I feel weak and shaky. Are there any side effects to this sort of pressure that may affect my diabetes?

In general, stress and worry tend to increase the blood glucose. One student told us that in the run up to her final examination, she had to double her insulin dose to keep perfect blood glucose control, even though she did not appear to her friends to be particularly anxious. Stress causes a release of adrenaline and other hormones, which antagonise the effect of insulin.

During periods of stress it may be difficult to keep to strict meal-times, so you could be at risk of going hypo. You should check your blood glucose and, if it is normal, you are simply experiencing the tiredness that we all feel after studying hard. Don't blame it on your diabetes but have an evening off from your studies.

HOSPITAL OPERATIONS

Recently, when I was in hospital to have my appendix removed, I was put on a 'sliding scale'. Please could you explain this, especially as it might save other people in a similar position from worrying?

The expression 'sliding scale' does sound rather alarming – but it is nothing to worry about. It can be difficult to predict exactly how much insulin someone will need during and after an operation, while they cannot eat or drink normally. The solution is to give glucose and insulin into a vein, with the dose of insulin adjusted depending on the blood glucose – known as a 'sliding scale'. More insulin is given if the level of blood glucose is high and this will have an immediate effect since it goes straight into the bloodstream. The blood glucose is usually checked every 1–2 hours and the insulin adjusted accordingly. In this way, diabetes control can be carefully regulated throughout the operation and until the person is eating again. Once this stage is reached, insulin may be given as three or four injections a day, the dose given at each injection being deter-mined from the amount of insulin required during the 'sliding scale' period.

Must I tell my dentist that I have diabetes and will this affect my treatment in any way?

Having diabetes will not affect your dental treatment. However, it is important to remove all possibility of a hypo while you are in the dentist's chair. If you are on insulin, warn your dentist that you cannot overrun a snack time or mealtime. It is less embarrassing to mention this before the start of a session than to have to munch glucose tablets while the dentist is trying to administer treatment. If your mouth is painful before or after your visit to the dentist, you may not be able to eat normal meals, which will require an adjustment in your insulin or tablets.

Obviously you must warn your dentist if you are due to have any form of heavy sedation. If someone on insulin is to have dental treatment needing a general anaesthetic, this is usually done in hospital.

Is someone with diabetes more likely to suffer from tooth decay or gum trouble?

There is an increased risk of infection in people whose diabetes is poorly controlled. The gums may become infected and this in turn may lead to tooth decay. However, someone who is well controlled is not prone to any particular dental problem – in fact, there is a positive advantage to avoiding sweets, which cause dental caries (tooth decay).

I have been told that, as I have diabetes, I don't have to pay for dental treatment. Is this true?

No. Dental treatment is not free to people who have diabetes. If you are entitled to benefits such as Income Support, you may be able to claim some help with the cost of treatment.

DRIVING

I drive a lot in my work and my lunchtime varies from day to day. Does this matter? I am on two injections of insulin a day.

This can be a problem. The twice-daily insulin regimen is designed to provide a boost of insulin at mid-day to cope with the lunchtime intake of food. Once the early morning injection of insulin has been given, there is no way of delaying the mid-day surge. It is very common for people who are well controlled on two injections a day to run a low blood sugar before lunch. Here are some possible solutions.

- Always check your blood glucose before driving, particularly if a meal is due. The DVLA now recommends this practice.

- Keep some food, such as biscuits or fruit, with you while driving so you can eat if your sugar goes low.

- Change to the basal bolus insulin regimen so that you have a small dose of short-acting insulin before each main meal with long-acting insulin in the evening to control your blood sugar overnight. If you use a short-acting analogue (such as NovoRapid® or Humalog®) you should not even need snacks between meals. However, we would still advise you to test before driving.

If I have diabetes, do I have to declare this when applying for a driving licence? If so, will I have to prove I am fit to drive?

Anyone whose diabetes is treated by diet alone does not need to inform the DVLA (Driving and Vehicle Licensing Agency). If your diabetes is treated by tablets or insulin, you must declare this when applying for a driving licence. If you already hold a driving licence, you must tell the DVLA as soon as you have been diagnosed.

When you have notified the DVLA, you will receive a form asking for details about your diabetes and the names of any doctors whom you see regularly. You will be asked to sign a declaration allowing your doctors to disclose medical details about your condition. There is usually no difficulty over someone with diabetes obtaining a licence to drive, though the bureaucracy may be irritating. The DVLA now advises people to test their blood glucose before driving, which is another cause of frustration but at least ensures that it is safe for you to drive.

If you are treated by tablets, you will be able to obtain an unrestricted licence, provided that you undertake to inform the DVLA of any change in your treatment or if you develop any complications of diabetes.

If you are treated by insulin, the licence will be valid for only three years instead of up to the age of 70, which is normal in the UK. It is the risk of sudden and severe hypoglycaemia which makes people liable to this form of discrimination. In general the only people who have difficulty in obtaining a licence are those on insulin with very erratic control and a history of hypos causing unconsciousness. Once their condition has been controlled and severe hypos abolished, they can reapply for a licence with confidence.

Diabetes UK has successfully campaigned for regulations on C1 licences to be changed. Previously, blanket restrictions were imposed on insulin users wishing to drive small vans and lorries between 3.5 and 7.5 tonnes. The revised regulations enable anyone taking insulin to be individually assessed on their fitness to drive, even if they have previously had their entitlement withdrawn. Restrictions on other Group 2 vehicles (heavier vehicles and passenger-carrying vehicles, such as minibuses) remain. For more information, contact Diabetes UK.

When I was filling out a form for the DVLA, one of the questions asked whether I had had laser treatment in both eyes. Why do the DVLA need this information?

The DVLA may ask you to have a 'visual fields test' if you have had laser treatment in both eyes, and your licence will be revoked if you cannot pass this test. The reason behind this is that in a few cases, very heavy laser therapy can reduce the field of vision – making it like looking through a keyhole. If you are having a visual fields test, you should have the type in which both eyes are tested at the same time. This test is the DVLA driving standard.

Do I have to inform my insurance company that I have diabetes?

When applying for motor insurance, you must declare that you have diabetes. Failure to disclose this can invalidate your cover if you need to make a claim. The Disability Discrimination Act 1996 outlawed the charging of higher premiums for groups of people where no higher risk rate has been proven, as is the case with diabetes. Unfortunately, there are some companies that still discriminate, but Diabetes UK Services has arranged a car insurance scheme to help make life easier. (See Appendix 2 for more information.)

I have heard that a driver who had a motor accident while hypo was successfully prosecuted for driving under the influence of drugs and heavily fined. As someone who takes insulin I was horrified to hear this verdict.

Several people on insulin have been charged with this offence after a hypo at the wheel when the only 'drug' that they have used is insulin. It may seem very unfair but, for any victim of such an accident, it is no consolation that the person responsible was hypo rather than under the influence of illegal drugs or alcohol. These cases emphasise the importance of taking driving seriously.

The rules for driving are:

- Always check your blood glucose before driving;
- If it is low, eat or take a glucose drink before you drive;
- Always carry food in your car and have some immediately if you feel warning of a hypo;
- If you think you may be hypo, pull off the road immediately, stop the car, turn off the ignition and remove the key;
- Do not resume driving until you are sure your blood glucose is in the normal range.

I have been a bus driver for 15 years and was found to have diabetes five years ago. Up until now I have been on tablets but may need to go onto insulin. Does this mean I will lose my job?

As a bus driver you will hold a PCV (Passenger Carrying Vehicle) licence. People on insulin are not allowed to drive a PCV. You are faced with a very difficult choice – either to continue on tablets feeling unwell but holding down your job, or else to start insulin and feel much better, but lose your source of employment. We would have to advise you to go onto insulin as you will need this eventually anyway and if your blood glucose is high for a prolonged period you risk long-term complications.

Holders of a LGV (Large Goods Vehicle) licence will also lose their licence and thus their livelihood if insulin treatment is to be started. LGV drivers who have been on insulin *since before 1991 and held their HGV licence since then* may keep their licence provided that they can prove that their control of their diabetes is good and they are not subject to hypos.

I have worked as a bus driver all my working life. I first got diabetes five years ago and have been well controlled till about six months ago. My doctor tells me that tablets are no longer working and that I must go onto insulin. This means I will lose my job, my source of income and probably my house.

This tragic situation is all too common. Some people in your situation have no difficulty in finding another way of earning money and paying the mortgage. However, others find it hard to give up their driving and believe no other job will match their present salary. There is no easy solution when you are faced with deciding between your health and your job. The choice becomes easier if you are feeling unwell, perhaps with symptoms of high sugars such as thirst and tiredness. We know some people in your situation who feel perfectly fit and cannot believe that there is a problem with their health. This makes their decision particularly difficult as they have to take their doctor's word that they need to have insulin.

I recently read a newspaper article that implied that people with diabetes who are breathalysed can produce a positive reading even though they have not been drinking alcohol. What does this mean?

Diabetes has no effect on breathalyser tests for alcohol even if acetone is present on the breath. However, the Lion Alcolmeter, widely used by the police, does also measure ketones, though this does not interfere with the alcohol measurement. Anyone breathalysed by the police may also be told that they have ketones and that they should consult their own doctor. These ketones may be caused either by diabetes that is out of control or by a long period of fasting.

ALCOHOL

My husband likes a pint of beer in the evening. He has now been found to have diabetes and has to stick to a diet. Does this mean he will have to give up drinking beer?

No. He can still drink beer but, if he is trying to lose weight, he will need to reduce his overall calorie intake and, unfortunately, all alcohol contains calories. There are about 180 calories in a pint of beer and this is equivalent to a large bread roll. Special 'diabetic' lager contains less carbohydrate but more alcohol so in the end it contains the same number of calories, with the drawback of being more expensive and more potent. He should probably also avoid the 'strong' brews, which are often labelled as being low in carbohydrate, as these are higher in alcohol and calories than the ordinary types of beer and lager. Low-alcohol and alcohol-free beers and lagers often contain a lot of sugar, so, if he decides to change to these, he should look for the ones also labelled as being low in sugar.

Overall your husband is probably better off drinking ordinary beer, but if he is overweight he should restrict the amount he drinks.

My partner has just been changed from tablets to insulin for his diabetes. He has been told that if he drinks alcohol, his blood sugar may go low. We had always thought that beer caused the blood sugar to rise. What should he do when he next goes out with his friends?

It is certainly true that beer can cause an initial rise in the blood glucose since it contains a lot of carbohydrate. However, alcohol itself has a direct effect on the liver which prevents it from releasing glucose when the blood glucose falls. This usually happens several hours later and may result in a hypo the following morning.

The overall effect of a particular alcoholic drink depends on the proportion of alcohol to carbohydrate. For instance, lemonade shandy (high carbohydrate, low alcohol) will have a different effect on the blood glucose from vodka and diet tonic (low carbohydrate, high alcohol). 'Diabetic' lager is more likely than ordinary beer to cause a hypo because it contains less carbohydrate but more alcohol.

To counteract the glucose-lowering effect of alcohol, it may be sensible for your partner to eat a sandwich or cereal and milk to provide extra carbohydrate before going to bed. He may also need to reduce his pre-breakfast insulin.

> *I believe that it is dangerous to drink alcohol if certain tablets are being taken. Does this apply to tablets used in diabetes?*

In general, no. However, alcohol may alter the response to a hypo (this has been discussed in the previous question) and some tablets used for diabetes can cause hypos. The most widely used are sulphonylureas (see Table 2.7). If you are taking a sulphonylurea and are going to drink alcohol, you should be aware of the possibility of a hypo. In practice this is very uncommon.

> *I've heard that there is evidence that a moderate amount of alcohol is part of a healthy diet, and that it reduces the risk of heart disease and strokes. My dietitian made me cut down my alcohol intake to one glass of wine a day, which is much less than I used to drink. What should I do?*

Recent research shows that alcohol in moderation reduces the risk of heart attacks, strokes and premature death in people with diabetes (or without); indeed the effects may be even more impressive in people with diabetes. Our view is that moderate alcohol intake (up to a maximum of half a bottle of wine a day, or equivalent) should be encouraged, but within a calorie-regulated diet, if you are overweight.

DRUGS

My son was told that people with diabetes should not use Betnovate cream because it contains steroids. Is this true and why?

It is best to avoid using powerful steroid creams such as Betnovate unless there is a serious skin condition. Very often a weak steroid preparation or some bland ointment is just as effective in clearing up mild patches of eczema and other rashes. Unfortunately, too often the very strong steroids are used first, instead of as a last resort. These strong steroids can be absorbed into the body through the skin and lead to a number of unwanted side effects. This applies to all people with skin problems and not just people with diabetes. One of the side effects of steroids is a rise in the blood glucose level. Thus, someone without diabetes may develop it while taking steroids and a person treated with diet only may need to go onto tablets or insulin.

If there are good medical reasons for your son to take steroids, in whatever form, he should test his blood for signs of poor control. If he is already taking insulin, the dose may need to be increased.

My wife suffers from bad indigestion. She is afraid to take indigestion tablets in case they upset her diabetes. Can you advise her what to do?

Indigestion tablets and medicines do not upset diabetes.

Is it safe to take water tablets with diabetes?

Water tablets (diuretics) are given to people who are retaining too much fluid in the body. This fluid retention may happen in heart failure and cause swelling of the ankles or shortness of breath. Diuretics are usually very effective but, as a side effect, they may cause a slight increase in the blood glucose. This is especially true of the milder diuretics from the thiazide group, such as Navidrex®.

The increase in glucose is only slight but can sometimes mean that someone with diabetes controlled by diet alone may need to take tablets. People already on insulin are not affected by diuretics. The thiazide group of tablets is also used in the treatment of raised blood pressure.

> *I have been on insulin for diabetes for seven years. I was recently found to have raised blood pressure and was given tablets, called beta-blockers, by my doctor. Since then I have had a bad hypo in which I collapsed without the normal warning signs of sweating, shaking, etc. Could the blood pressure tablets have caused this severe hypo?*

Beta-blockers are widely used for the treatment of high blood pressure and certain heart conditions. They have an 'anti-adrenaline' effect, which theoretically could damp down the normal 'adrenaline' response to a hypo (see the section *Hypos* in Chapter 3). However, research has shown that beta-blockers do not reduce the adrenaline warning of a hypo. Some beta-blockers have been designed to have their effect mainly on the heart without blocking the general adrenaline reaction. These selective beta-blockers, such as atenolol or bisoprolol, are theoretically safer for people taking insulin.

Is there any special cough mixture for people with diabetes?

There are various sugar-free cough mixtures that can be bought from your chemist. However, there is only a tiny bit of sugar in a dose of ordinary cough mixture and this amount will not have any appreciable effect on the level of blood glucose.

Please could you give me a list of tablets or medicines that may interfere with my diabetes?

The important medicines that affect diabetes have already been discussed in this section. There are no medicines that must never be used but the following might increase the blood glucose and upset your control:

- steroids (e.g. prednisolone, Betnovate® ointment, Becotide® inhaler) may cause a rise in blood glucose level but inhalers or ointment will only have this effect if taken in large doses;
- thiazide diuretics (e.g. bendroflumethiazide);
- the contraceptive pill;
- hormone replacement therapy;
- certain bronchodilators (e.g. Ventolin®) might have a slight effect of raising the blood glucose;
- growth hormone treatment.

SMOKING

When my doctor diagnosed diabetes, he told me to stop smoking. Could you tell me if there is a particular health hazard associated with smoking and diabetes? The problem is made worse for me by the fact that I have to lose weight and, if I stop smoking, I will do just the opposite.

Smoking is a danger, both to the lungs and because of the risk of increased arterial disease, which affects anyone who smokes. Someone with long-standing diabetes is at risk of problems with poor blood circulation, and it is unwise to increase this risk by continuing to smoke. If the discovery that you have diabetes has come as a nasty shock, you could turn it to your advantage and decide to make important changes in lifestyle, by eating less and giving up cigarettes. It may be a lot to ask, but many people manage to carry out this 'double'. It won't kill you – on the contrary, you may live longer.

There is a lot of support available now for people who want to give up smoking, and your GP or practice nurse should be able to offer you advice on whom to contact. They may run a group or clinic to help you quit. Some people are helped by nicotine gum or patches and we deal with these in a later question in this section.

Since my husband, who has had diabetes for 23 years, has stopped smoking, he has had high blood glucose tests. Why is this?

Your husband should be congratulated for giving up smoking. Most people who give up smoking put on weight, on average 4 kg (9 lb). This is because cigarettes suppress the appetite and make the body operate less efficiently, thus burning up more fuel (food). If your husband has put on weight, this explains his higher blood glucose levels. He should try to reduce weight to improve his diabetes. If he is already thin and his blood glucose levels are high then he will have to take tablets or insulin to get his diabetes under control.

My doctor has strongly advised me to give up smoking and suggested that I try nicotine patches. I was surprised to find that the information leaflet enclosed with the patches advised people with diabetes not to use the patches. Is this true?

It sounds as though the manufacturer is being overcautious. The main reason for giving up smoking is to reduce the damage that it does to the blood supply to the heart, brain and legs. With each cigarette smoked, the nicotine inhaled narrows the small blood vessels. This narrowing eventually becomes permanent, which explains why smoking increases the risk of heart attacks, strokes and gangrene. Nicotine patches have been shown to be a most effective way of helping people to stop smoking.

Nicotine has the same effect on the blood vessels whether from patches or from cigarettes. However, patches are no worse than cigarettes and, if they help you to give up smoking, the overall benefit will be enormous, especially with regard to your circulation. Don't be afraid to try nicotine patches in the recommended dose. The same advice applies to nicotine chewing gum and the newer nicotine inhaler.

PRESCRIPTION CHARGES AND SOCIAL SECURITY BENEFITS

I believe that people with diabetes are entitled to free prescriptions. Please could you tell me how to apply?

One of the few advantages of having diabetes is exemption from payment on all prescription charges – even for treatment unconnected with the diabetes itself. People treated on diet alone are not exempt from prescription charges.

You must obtain a form, called *NHS prescriptions – how to get them free*, from your GP. The completed form should be signed by your doctor who will send it to the Primary Care Trust (PCT). You will then receive an exemption certificate. Please remember to carry this certificate wherever you are likely to need a prescription, for example travelling in the UK. The certificate lasts for five years, and you will then need to renew it.

What Social Security benefits am I entitled to now that I have diabetes?

There are no special benefits given automatically to people with diabetes. You may claim Disability Living Allowance if you have a child with diabetes who is under the age of 12, and it may be possible to obtain this allowance for a child up to the age of 16 if you can prove that the child needs extra supervision and care. Diabetes

UK Careline can provide you with information to help you complete the necessary forms.

For more information about benefits, we suggest that you contact either Diabetes UK Careline, the Disability Alliance (addresses in Appendix 2), or the Benefits Agency. This organisation deals with Social Security benefits on behalf of the Department of Work and Pensions, and you can make enquiries either at its offices or by phone. You will find its addresses and telephone numbers (it has several freephone enquiry lines) in your local phone book under 'Benefits Agency'. From the homepage of the website www.direct.gov.uk you can go straight to 'money, tax and benefits'.

Since developing diabetes I have found that my food bills have risen alarmingly. Are there any special allowances that I can claim to offset the very high cost of the food?

Most people with diabetes are not entitled to any special allowance and, indeed, there is no real need for them to eat different food from others. Special diabetic products are not necessary. Now that people are encouraged to eat food that is high rather than low in carbohydrate, they do not have to fall back on expensive protein as a source of calories. There is a question in the *Diet* section of Chapter 2 offering suggestions on keeping down the cost of food (see p. 41).

My mother has had diabetes for 12 years and is subject to crashing hypos for no reason. She needs someone to be with her all the time. Would we be eligible for an Attendance Allowance as she needs watching 24 hours a day?

If you have to provide a continuous watch over your mother, you can apply for an Attendance Allowance. Before admitting defeat, however, it would be better to try every means of preventing the hypos. Presumably your mother is having insulin, though you do not mention the dose or type of insulin. It would be worth checking with the local diabetes service if anything could be done to reduce the frequency of hypos. Changing to more frequent but smaller doses of insulin might solve the problem. You may have to spend time and energy getting to grips with your mother's diabetes. It would do more for her self-confidence to abolish the hypos than to get an Attendance Allowance.

Sometimes people who are developing Alzheimer's disease are at risk of hypos because they forget to eat at the correct time. We have a patient who has overcome this by wearing a watch with a timer, which can be set to ring an alarm at mealtimes. One such device is called a MedicAlarm – see addresses in Appendix 2.

MISCELLANEOUS

Is there any objection to my donating blood? I am on two injections of soluble insulin a day and my general health is fine.

It is hard to understand why a fit person with diabetes should not be a blood donor. However, the blood transfusion authorities do not accept blood from people on insulin. They suggest that the antibodies to insulin found in all people having injections may in some way harm the recipient of the blood.

Is it true that someone with diabetes should not use an electric blanket?

It is perfectly safe for you to use an electric blanket, although most underblankets should be used only to warm up the bed in advance. The manufacturers usually recommend that underblankets should be switched off before you get into bed. However, there are now underblankets that can be left on all night on a very low heat and these would be safe to use, provided that you follow the manufacturer's instructions. Overblankets can be left on all night, but again you should always check the manufacturer's instructions.

Hot-water bottles are rather more dangerous as their temperature is not controlled. People with a slight degree of nerve damage can fail to realise that a bottle full of very hot water may be burning the skin of their feet. This is a recognised cause of foot ulcers. It is better to be safe than sorry and avoid the comfort of a hot-water bottle. Bedsocks are a possible alternative for cold feet, or you could try one of the small electric heating pads now on the market. Again you need to be careful how you use these and follow the manufacturer's instructions – not all of them are suitable for use in bed.

Is it safe for people with diabetes to use sunbeds and saunas?

It is as safe as for those without diabetes: exposure to ultraviolet radiation is known to increase the risk of skin cancer. If you do use one, make sure that you can recognise the signs of a hypo when you are hot and sweaty. Keep some means of treating a hypo with you – not with your clothes in the changing room.

I have diabetes and would dearly love to have my ears pierced but, when I asked my doctor about this, he said there was a chance that my ears would swell. Please could you advise me if there is a great risk of this happening?

Anyone who has their ears pierced runs a small risk of infection until the wound heals completely. The risk in a person with well controlled diabetes is no higher than normal. If your ears do become red, swollen and painful, you may need an antibiotic.

Is there any connection between vertigo and diabetes? I have had diabetes for just over two years controlled on diet alone.

Vertigo, in the strict medical sense, describes the sensation when the world seems to be spinning round. It is usually due to disease of the inner ear or of the part of the brain that controls balance. This is not connected with diabetes in any way. However, simple dizzy spells are a common problem with many possible causes, which may be difficult to diagnose. If dizziness occurs when you move from sitting down to standing, it may be the result of a sudden fall in blood pressure. This can sometimes be due to a loss of reflexes as a result of diabetic neuropathy (see Chapter 8: **Long-term complications** for more information about neuropathy). There are no other connections between diabetes and vertigo.

My husband's grandmother is 84 and has diabetes. Although she is fiercely independent, she cannot look after herself properly and will have to go into a residential home. Can you let me know of any homes that cater especially for people with diabetes?

B ecause diabetes is becoming increasingly common in the elderly, the staff in most residential homes are experienced in looking after people with diabetes. They will probably be happy to do urine tests, ensure that diet is satisfactory and see that she gets her tablets and, if necessary, insulin injections.

My wife, who developed diabetes a few weeks ago, is about to return to work. I feel that she should wear some sort of identity disc or bracelet showing that she has diabetes but she is reluctant to wear anything too eye-catching. Have you any suggestions?

I t is very important that all people with diabetes, especially those on insulin, should wear some form of identification. Accidents do happen and it may be vital for any medical emergency team to know that your wife has diabetes.

Medic-Alert provides stainless steel bracelets or necklets which are functional if not very beautiful. They can also be obtained in silver, gold plate, and 9-carat gold. Medic-Alert's address is in Appendix 2.

SOS/Talisman (address is in Appendix 2) produces a medallion which can be unscrewed to reveal identification and medical details.

These can be bought in most jewellers and come in a wide range of styles and prices, including some in 9-carat gold. Other products are always coming on to the market, and *Balance*, the magazine produced by Diabetes UK, usually carries advertisements.

I recently enquired about having electrolysis treatment for excess hair. I was told that, as I had diabetes, I would need a letter from my doctor stating that my diabetes did not encourage hair growth. Could I use wax hair removers instead?

There is no objection to your having electrolysis. Diabetes does not cause excessive hair growth. It sounds as though the firm doing the electrolysis is being overcautious.

People with diabetes can use the same methods of hair removal as those without diabetes – no special precautions are needed.

Could you tell me what ointment to use for skin irritation?

The most common cause of skin irritation in people with diabetes is itching around the genital region (pruritus vulvae). The most important treatment is to eliminate glucose from the urine by controlling diabetes. However, the itching can be relieved temporarily by cream containing a fungicide (e.g. nystatin).

I have recently been given a foot spa and was surprised to see a caution on the side of the box that it is not suitable for people with diabetes. Is this true?

If you have neuropathy (nerve damage), you should check with your diabetes team before using the spa. If you don't have neuropathy, make sure that you check the temperature of the water carefully and don't soak your feet for too long as this will make the skin soggy, easily damaged and prone to infection.

6 | Sex, contraception and HRT

These days there is a more relaxed attitude to discussing subjects such as sex and contraception, but many people still find it difficult to ask questions about these topics. Generally, people with diabetes are no different from those without diabetes in any aspect of sexuality, fertility, infertility and contraception. However, there are some problems, such as the increased risk of impotence (sometimes known as erectile dysfunction) in men who have had diabetes for many years. This is often caused by neuropathy (nerve damage) or poor blood supply. Nowadays there are a variety of treatments available and if you are concerned about erectile dysfunction you should speak to your doctor. There have been very few studies of the effect of diabetes on sexual function in women but there is some evidence to suggest that women who have had diabetes for many years may have more difficulty achieving orgasm.

Various contraceptive devices have at times been said to be less effective in women with diabetes – the evidence for this is poor and women with diabetes should choose their contraception depending on their personal preferences. Some oral contraceptive pills may be more suitable than others but your doctor will be able to advise you. Oral contraceptives do not increase the risk of developing diabetes.

IMPOTENCE (ERECTILE DYSFUNCTION)

I am a happily married man and have been diagnosed with diabetes. I have been told that diabetes could affect my sex life. Is this correct?

The majority of people with diabetes, both male and female, lead a completely normal and full sex life. It is true that problems may occur but many of these have nothing to do with diabetes. If your blood glucose levels are consistently high, this could affect your sex life. Some men have either nerve damage or arterial disease causing loss of sexual potency (erectile dysfunction), which can be directly attributed to diabetes.

Is it normal for people with diabetes to suddenly find themselves totally uninterested in sexual intercourse? My husband is really upset about my lack of desire!

The feeling that you describe is more common in women than men, but is no more likely in women with diabetes. Anything which makes you tired can lead to loss of interest in sex and poorly controlled diabetes can certainly affect your energy levels. In these circumstances loss of interest in sex is one of casualties of the high blood sugar.

I have had erratic blood glucose levels recently. Would low blood glucose affect my ability to achieve or maintain an erection and more importantly, my ability to ejaculate?

Not unless the blood glucose is very low (less than 4 mmol/L), in which case many aspects of brain and nerve function are affected and this could reduce both your potency and ability to ejaculate. These will return to normal when your blood glucose is stable.

Am I likely to become impotent? I have had diabetes for five years.

There is no doubt that many men with diabetes worry about the possibility of developing erectile dysfunction (impotence) in the future. Our advice is to try to keep your diabetes under good control and this will reduce the risk of future complications. If you are unlucky enough to develop erectile difficulties, there are now a number of treatments available to help. Your doctor will be able to advise you and if necessary refer you to a specialist clinic.

My husband, who is middle-aged with Type 2 diabetes, has been impotent for the past two years. Please will you explain what causes this?

Erectile dysfunction (impotence) worries many people and occurs in men with and without diabetes. It appears that one in five men with diabetes may develop this problem at some stage in their lives, though the condition may be reversible. Most men with erectile difficulties do not have diabetes and a number of other factors such as anxiety, depression, overwork, tiredness, stress, alcohol excess and grief can cause this problem. Any man may find that he is temporarily impotent and fear of failure can make things worse. Overwork or worry can lead to lack of interest in sex and erectile dysfunction. Excess alcohol, while not causing lack of interest in sex, may lead to impotence.

Some men with diabetes do develop erectile difficulties, as a result of problems with the blood supply or the nerve supply to the penis. This usually develops slowly and in younger people it can often be prevented by strict blood glucose control. Treatments such as Viagra® are now available and can be prescribed by your husband's doctor. In older people the condition is more difficult to treat successfully, partly because there may be other medical factors in addition to diabetes. Your husband should discuss the matter further with his own doctor.

Recently, I have had trouble keeping an erection – has this anything to do with my diabetes? I also had a vasectomy a few years ago.

This is difficult to answer without knowing more about you and your medical history. Vasectomy may lead to impotence for psychological reasons but is unlikely to have caused any damage which might affect erections. Failure to maintain an adequate erection may be an early sign of diabetic neuropathy and you might need blood tests to rule out other medical causes. However, it is often a symptom of overwork or simply the ageing process.

I have been impotent for months. Is there some drug or hormone that will help me?

It is rare for a hormonal abnormality to cause impotence although it is normal practice to check the hormone levels by a blood test in any man with erectile dysfunction. If your impotence is caused by a hormonal deficiency, treatment with the replacement hormone (testosterone) may cure the problem. It is essential to get a correct diagnosis in order to ensure appropriate therapy. Many cases of impotence are due to psychological causes and often respond to appropriate advice or to drug treatment. Injecting a drug called Caverject® directly into the penis can sometimes be helpful. It leads to an immediate erection and the result is often good enough to make this an acceptable form of therapy.

Viagra® is the first oral treatment for impotence to be licensed in the UK. It works by helping to relax the blood vessels in the penis, allowing more blood to flow into the penis causing an erection, and will only be effective if the man is sexually stimulated. It is available on the NHS, but officially the amount is limited to four tablets a month. It is important to use the full strength (100 mg) as lower amounts are much less likely to work. Viagra does have some strange side effects which you should ask about when it is prescribed.

I suffered a stroke affecting the right side of my body 12 months ago at the age of 40 and now suffer from partial impotence. The onset seemed to coincide not with the stroke but with taking anticoagulants. Are these known to cause impotence? I have also heard that blood pressure tablets can cause impotence and I have been taking these for three months. Could this be a factor?

A severe stroke can sometimes lead to impotence. A stroke is often due to narrowing of the arteries inside the head and the arteries elsewhere may also be narrowed. If those supplying blood to the penis are affected, this could contribute to your erectile dysfunction. You are also quite right about the drugs. Some blood pressure lowering drugs may cause impotence and can interfere with ejaculation. It would be unwise to stop taking the drugs since this would lead to loss of control of your blood pressure and the risk of a further stroke. However, there is individual variation in the way people respond to different tablets and you could ask your doctor if there are any alternative blood pressure tablets you could try. Anticoagulant tablets are not known to cause impotence.

I have heard about weekend Viagra. Could you tell me more?

One of the drawbacks with Viagra® is that it only has its effect from one to three hours after taking the tablet. This may take much of the spontaneity out of sex. A newer tablet called Cialis® starts to have effect in 30 minutes and lasts for 12 hours more – as the manufacturer claims, 'for the best part of a weekend'. Levitra® is another drug similar to Viagra which should be taken 25–60 minutes before you want to have sex.

I have heard that Viagra may be dangerous and cause heart attacks. Is this true?

Apart from the obvious answer about sex and heart attacks, Viagra and the other drugs in the same group do not normally have a bad effect on the heart – in fact Viagra was first developed as a drug to help heart disease. There is one very important occasion when Viagra may be dangerous for people with angina. If they are taking any form of nitrate, including a nitrate (GTN) spray, they should not take Viagra as this may cause sudden collapse. Commonly used nitrates are Suscard®, isosorbide and Imdur®. If you think you may be taking a nitrate for angina, please check with your doctor before taking Viagra. Since nitrates prevent angina, it is not really safe to stop taking them in order to be able to have sex stimulated by Viagra.

I have used Viagra for three years for impotence. At first it worked very well but the effect now seems to be wearing off. Is there anything else I can try?

There is another drug on the market, which is designed to help men achieve an erection. It is called apomorphine (or Uprima®), and should be placed under the tongue about 20 minutes before you want to have sex. Apomorphine has about the same success rate as Viagra, but may help some men who do not respond to Viagra. Apomorphine seems to be a safe drug, but you should avoid it if you have severe heart problems or if your blood pressure is low.

Is there any other treatment for impotence apart from Viagra?

Counselling by a therapist trained in this subject can be helpful, particularly in cases where the stresses and conflicts of life are the root cause. Testosterone should help men with a deficiency of this hormone. Vacuum therapy, with a device that looks like a rigid condom, can be very successful but does require a sense of humour in both partners. Injections of papaverine or alprostadil (Caverject®) into the penis, and penile implants (which require an operation) are also effective. Choosing the best option for you as a couple requires a considerable amount of thought and discussion, both with your partner and your doctor. In our experience, most partners are sympathetic and understanding about impotence (whatever the cause) if you can talk about it openly. Many diabetes departments hold special clinics for treatment of impotence and they prefer both partners to take part in the discussion.

After sexual intercourse I recently suffered quite a bad hypo. Is this likely to happen again and if so, what can be done to prevent it?

Like any physical activity, sex can lower the blood glucose and lead to hypoglycaemia. When this happens, and it is not at all uncommon, you need to deal with the hypo in the usual way using fruit juice or Lucozade (see section *Hypos* in Chapter 3). You may find it useful to keep some quick-acting carbohydrate close at hand.

CONTRACEPTION AND VASECTOMY

I have diabetes and want to start on the Pill. Are there any extra risks that women with diabetes run in using it?

The oral contraceptive pill is as effective for women with diabetes as for those without diabetes. It is now well known that the Pill carries a small risk of venous thrombosis, sometimes called DVT or deep vein thrombosis (where a vein becomes blocked by a blood clot) and pulmonary embolus (where the blood clot moves to the lung). To keep these risks to a minimum, you should take the smallest possible dose of oestrogen and your doctor will be able to advise you about the most suitable preparation. Some women are at higher risk and this includes those with a previous history of DVT or pulmonary embolus, smokers over the age of 35 years and those at high risk of stroke or heart attack. This last group includes women with a family history of heart disease or stroke at an early age and those with a high cholesterol or high blood pressure.

In general there is no reason why women with diabetes should not take the Pill, but if you have complications of diabetes such as high blood pressure, high cholesterol or kidney disease you may be at greater risk and you should consider an alternative method of contraception. The risk involved in pregnancy itself is greater than that of the Pill, so if you decide that the Pill is not for you it is important that you choose an effective alternative. Women with uncomplicated diabetes may certainly use the Pill and there are no additional risks.

When women with diabetes start using the Pill there is sometimes a slight deterioration of control. This is rarely a problem and is usually easily dealt with by a small increase in treatment, which in those taking insulin may mean a small increase in the dose. It is a simple matter to monitor the blood and make appropriate adjustments.

My doctor prescribed the Pill for me but on the packet it states that it is unsuitable for people with diabetes. As my doctor knows that I have diabetes is it safe enough for me?

There used to be some confusion about whether the Pill was suitable for women with diabetes but there is now general agreement that as long as there are no diabetes complications, they may use the Pill for contraceptive purposes without any increased risks compared with those who do not have diabetes. If you do have any diabetes-related complications you should speak to your doctor.

I want to try the progesterone-only contraceptive pill. Is it suitable for women with diabetes?

Yes, although this type of Pill has a higher failure rate than the combined pill so it has become less popular.

I have just started the menopause and wondered if I have to wait two years after my last period before doing away with contraception.

Although periods may become irregular and infrequent at the start of the menopause, it is still possible to be fertile, and this advice is a precaution against unwanted pregnancy. It applies equally to women with or without diabetes.

Can you please give me any information regarding vasectomy and any side effects it may have for men with diabetes?

Vasectomy is a relatively minor surgical procedure, which involves cutting and tying off the vas deferens – the tube that carries sperm from the testes to the penis. Vasectomy may be carried out under either local or general anaesthetic usually as a day case. It would be simpler to have it under local anaesthetic as this will not disturb the balance of your diabetes. The main side effect of the operation is discomfort, which may last for a few days although infections and other complications do rarely occur.

There are a few medical reasons for avoiding this operation but they apply equally to men without diabetes as they do to men with diabetes and your doctor will be able to discuss these with you.

I have diabetes and I am marrying a man with diabetes in eight weeks' time. Please could you advise me on how to stop becoming pregnant?

We are not quite clear whether you wish to be sterilised and never have children or whether you are seeking contraceptive advice. If you and your fiancé have decided that you do not want to have the anxiety of your children inheriting diabetes and have made a clear decision not to have children, you have the option of your fiancé having a vasectomy or being sterilised yourself.

These are very fundamental decisions and will require careful thought because they are probably best considered as irreversible procedures. If you are quite certain about not having children, we would advise you both to discuss this with your GP and seek referral either to a surgeon for vasectomy for your fiancé or to a gynaecologist for sterilisation. Whichever you decide, you must both attend since no surgeon will undertake this procedure without being convinced that you have thought about it carefully and have come to a clear, informed decision.

If our interpretation of your question has not been right and you are simply looking for contraceptive advice, then the best source of this is either your GP or local family planning clinic. All the usual forms of contraceptives are suitable for women with diabetes, so it is just a question of discovering which best suits you and your partner.

I have been warned that IUDs are more unreliable in women with diabetes. Is this really true?

IUDs (intrauterine contraceptive devices) are generally regarded as slightly less reliable contraceptives than the Pill, and there has been one report suggesting they may be even less reliable when used by women with diabetes. No other studies have backed up this observation. There has also been a report suggesting that women with diabetes may be slightly more susceptible to pelvic infections when using an IUD. On balance, we believe that IUDs should be considered effective and useful in women with diabetes.

THRUSH

I suffer with thrush. My diabetes has been well controlled for ten years now. I do regular blood tests and most of them are less than 10 mmol/L and, whenever I check a urine test, it is always negative. I have been taking the oral contraceptive pill for three years and I understand that both diabetes and the Pill can lead to thrush. Can you advise me what to do?

Since your diabetes is well controlled and your urine consistently free from glucose, diabetes can probably be ruled out as a cause of the thrush. It sounds as if you are either being reinfected by your partner or alternatively it is an uncommon side effect of the Pill, and you should discuss the need for a change of contraception with your doctor.

I keep getting recurrence of vaginal thrush and my doctor says that, as I have diabetes, there is nothing that I can do about this – is this correct?

Thrush is due to an infection with a yeast (*Candida*) that thrives in the presence of a lot of glucose. If your diabetes is badly controlled and you are passing a lot of glucose in your urine, you will be very susceptible to vaginal thrush and, however much ointment and cream you use, it is likely to recur. The best treatment is to control your diabetes so well that there is no glucose in your urine, but if the thrush persists, you will need antifungal treatment from your doctor. If you keep your urine free from glucose, you should stay free from further thrush infections.

HORMONE REPLACEMENT THERAPY (HRT)

Can you tell me if hormone replacement therapy for the menopause is suitable for women with diabetes?

Hormone replacement therapy (HRT) for the menopause consists of small doses of oestrogen and progesterone given to replace the hormones normally produced by the ovaries. Oestrogen levels in the blood begin to fall at the menopause and, if this happens rapidly, it can cause unpleasant symptoms, such as hot flushes. Replacement therapy is designed to allow a more gradual decline in the female hormones. There has been a lot of publicity about the adverse effects of HRT in the last few years and there is some evidence to suggest an increased risk of breast cancer, thrombosis and stroke. However, these risks have to be balanced against the benefits of HRT. The evidence shows that for every 1000 women taking combined oestrogen and progestogen replacement therapy for five years, there will be:

- six extra cases of breast cancer;
- nine extra cases of thrombosis (blood clots) in the legs or in the lungs;
- two extra cases of stroke.

Women with diabetes already have an increased risk of stroke and heart attack and HRT may increase this. The current advice is that women with severe menopausal symptoms benefit from short-term HRT but for those without symptoms the risks outweigh the benefits. In the past, HRT has been recommended for prevention of osteoporosis but since it may be responsible for the unwanted side effects listed above, some experts recommend that other preventative treatments are used in preference to HRT.

These are not easy decisions but doctors are now cautious about recommending HRT routinely to all women. As the risks of stroke are greater for women with diabetes, we would advise that HRT is only used by women with severe menopausal symptoms, and for as short a period as possible.

I want to try and avoid osteoporosis by taking HRT. As I have diabetes, is this sensible?

HRT is the most effective treatment for the prevention of osteoporosis but because of the problems mentioned in the previous question, some doctors are cautious about recommending it as a first choice. The decision depends on your individual risk of developing osteoporosis. If you have a high risk, you may choose to take HRT and accept the small chance of unwanted complications; if your risk is low, you may prefer to try an alternative, which may be less effective but lessen your chances of complications. Please speak to your doctor about this. You should, of course, take general measures such as ensuring adequate calcium in your diet and taking regular weight-bearing exercise.

Are the patch forms of HRT as suitable for women with diabetes as the tablets?

There is no known difference between tablets and patches; all the answers to the questions above apply equally to patches.

TERMINATION OF PREGNANCY

I have become pregnant and really don't want a baby at the moment. Is diabetes grounds for termination of pregnancy?

No, not unless your doctor considers that the pregnancy would be detrimental to your health, which may sometimes be the case if you have complications of diabetes. If you do not have any complications the reasons for termination of pregnancy apply equally to women with and without diabetes.

I am going into hospital for an abortion. I am worried that the doctors might not do it as I have diabetes. Should I have told someone?

There is no added hazard for women with diabetes who undergo termination of pregnancy, and care of the diabetes during this operation does not raise any special difficulties. It is still important to tell your gynaecologist that you have diabetes so that good control can be maintained during this time.

FERTILITY

I have recently got married and my wife and I are keen to start a family. Are people with diabetes more likely to be infertile?

There is nothing to suggest that men with diabetes are any less fertile than men who do not have diabetes and in general this is also true for women. However, women with consistently high blood glucose readings may find it more difficult to conceive. This may be a good thing as there is sound evidence to show that the outcome of pregnancy is much worse in women who conceive when their control is poor.

I have been trying for a baby for years and we have now decided to go for fertility counselling and possible treatment. Can people with diabetes expect the same treatment for infertility as people without?

Yes. As mentioned in the previous question, diabetes is rarely the cause of infertility. If control is anything other than excellent, improving control, aiming for an HbA$_{1c}$ of less than 7.5% should be the first goal. Referral to an infertility expert is the next step but good control would be necessary before treatment could be started.

I have told that I have PCOS and my doctor says this might make it difficult for me to conceive and also puts me at risk of developing diabetes. Could you explain this.

Polycystic ovary syndrome (PCOS) is a condition in which the ovaries have multiple small cysts that interfere with function and may upset the normal hormone balance, causing irregular periods. This can lead to reduced fertility. PCOS is often associated with being overweight and can lead to an increase in body hair. It is also linked with insulin resistance and an increased risk of developing type 2 diabetes. There are a number of possible treatments but in the past few years, metformin has been identified as an effective treatment which may increase fertility and reduce body hair.

7 | Pregnancy

Pregnancy was the first condition associated with diabetes where it was proved that poor blood glucose control led to complications for both mother and child and that these complications could be avoided by strict blood glucose control. The outcome for pregnant women with diabetes, and for their babies, is directly related to how well they control their blood glucose throughout the pregnancy. If control is good from the moment of conception to delivery, the risks to mother and baby can be little greater than in women without diabetes.

We now know that poor control at conception, when the egg is fertilised, can affect the way in which the egg divides and develops into the fetus (the stage at which all organs and limbs are present in minute form). This sometimes leads to congenital abnormalities such as spina bifida, hole in the heart and cleft palate. The risk of this happening can be reduced to a minimum, and possibly eliminated, by ensuring a normal HbA_{1c} before becoming pregnant. The evidence suggests that the higher the HbA_{1c} at conception, the higher the risk of an abnormality in the baby.

Some of these problems may be detected by ultrasound scan early in pregnancy, and termination may be considered if a major defect is found. If the scan shows a normal fetus, the outcome of the pregnancy will still be affected by the mother's blood glucose control during the rest of her pregnancy. Poor control tends to lead to big babies and this can be a problem for both mother and baby at the time of delivery. Sadly, there is also a greater risk of stillbirth in babies of mothers with poor diabetes control but careful monitoring of the baby close to the time of delivery has greatly reduced this risk.

A recent audit of pregnancy in mothers with diabetes (CEMACH – Confidential Enquiry into Maternal and Child Health) has come up with some disappointing results. In the course of this national audit, information was collected from all 231 maternity units in England, Wales and Northern Ireland, and showed that despite increasing awareness of the need for good control, the results for pregnancies complicated by diabetes are still very unsatisfactory. Babies of mothers with diabetes are:

- five times more likely to be stillborn;
- twice as likely to have a congenital malformation;
- twice as likely to weigh more than 4 kg (9 lb).

This is true for both Type 1 and Type 2 diabetes. See the website: www.cemach.org.uk/publications for full details.

These figures are very disturbing and compare unfavourably with other countries, such as Australia. There is clearly need for improvement since we know that with careful attention to diabetes control and close monitoring of the baby, the outcome of the pregnancy can be much better.

Modern antenatal care is usually shared between the diabetes specialist and the obstetrician, preferably at a joint clinic. Admission to hospital is rarely necessary as long as the pregnancy progresses normally and control remains good, in which case the pregnancy should continue close to its natural term. Any antenatal complications will be treated in the same way as they would be in women without diabetes. Once spontaneous labour begins, the only difference from the normal process is the need to keep the mother's blood glucose normal to prevent hypoglycaemia in the baby after delivery. Although the aim should always be for a normal delivery, mothers with diabetes do have a higher chance of needing a Caesarean section, particularly if the baby is large or needs to be delivered early.

Most women are able to make the great effort required to keep tight control during pregnancy but it is very difficult to keep this up once they are faced with the demands of a new baby and the need to avoid hypoglycaemia.

A very comprehensive pregnancy magazine is available from Diabetes UK.

PREPREGNANCY

The man I am going to marry has Type 2 diabetes.
Will any children we may have be at risk of diabetes?

Type 2 diabetes certainly runs in families and your children would be at risk of developing this later in life. Although this type of diabetes generally occurs in adults, you may have seen publicity about Type 2 diabetes affecting children. This is most likely to occur if the child is overweight and you can reduce the risk by encouraging healthy eating and an active lifestyle.

There is a rare form of Type 2 diabetes in which there is a strong hereditary tendency. This is called maturity onset diabetes of the young, commonly known as MODY. Were you or your fiancé to have this, the risk of your children getting diabetes of this unusual kind would be rather high. It is often a relatively mild form of diabetes and runs true to type throughout the generations.

The study of inheritance of diabetes is a complicated subject and you would be well advised to discuss this further with your specialist or a professional genetic counsellor.

*I am worried that, if I become pregnant while my husband's
diabetes is uncontrolled, the child will suffer – am I right?*

No. There is no known way in which poor control of your
husband's diabetes can affect the development of your child.

*I am 29 years old and have Type 2 diabetes. My husband
and I plan to start a family but first I would like to complete
a three-year degree course at university. By the time this
finishes I will be 32. Can you tell me if I shall then be too old
to have a baby?*

There is a trend nowadays for women to delay starting a family
until they are well into their thirties. Thirty-two is not too old
to have a child but if you have diabetes, there are some advantages
in having children earlier rather than later. The main reason for
this is that the longer you have had diabetes, the greater the risk of
developing complications, which may have a significant effect on the
pregnancy.

Having said this, many women with diabetes have successful pregnancies in their thirties and even forties. It is difficult to give exact
personal advice to individual people and the right person to talk to is
your family doctor or diabetes specialist, who will know both you and
your diabetes.

*I have diabetes treated by tablets, which I chose to take
rather than insulin, and I want to become pregnant. I have
had a previous miscarriage and am worried about the chance
of this happening again. Both my husband and I smoke and
enjoy the occasional glass of wine. How can I make sure that
this pregnancy is successful?*

The control of your diabetes will certainly affect the outcome of your
pregnancy – better control leads to more a successful pregnancy.
As you are planning your pregnancy, you can make sure that you

establish good control before conception. Your control is probably best maintained either by diet alone or, if this fails, by diet with insulin. Until recently, we did not advise women to take tablets for diabetes but there is now evidence to suggest that metformin is safe and does not affect the baby. So if you are taking metformin you can continue to take it but none of the other tablets used to treat type 2 diabetes are regarded as safe during pregnancy. If your diabetes can be controlled by metformin alone, that is fine, but you will need to stop any other tablets and that could mean that you need to change to insulin. You should discuss this with your doctor or nurse. As pregnancy progresses, an increasing amount of insulin is required to keep the blood glucose normal and even if you have been well controlled on metformin in the past, it is likely that insulin injections will be necessary at some stage. The most important thing is to make sure your diabetes is well controlled before you become pregnant and if your HbA_{1c} is above 6.5% on metformin you should consider starting insulin.

You obviously know already that smoking affects the baby and that heavy smoking is associated with more miscarriages and smaller babies. We suspect that you already know the answers to your question – you need to take insulin and give up smoking.

There is also more recent evidence to link even modest regular alcohol intake in pregnancy with an unfavourable outcome as far as the baby is concerned, so we suggest that you should stop drinking alcohol until the pregnancy is over.

Why must I ensure that my diabetes control is perfect during pregnancy?

This is to ensure that you reduce the risks to yourself and your baby to an absolute minimum. If you are able to achieve this degree of control from before the time of conception through to the time of delivery, the risks to your baby are only slightly greater than those for babies born to women without diabetes. On the other hand, if your diabetes is poorly controlled, the risk to your baby increases dramatically.

I have Type 2 diabetes and am thinking of a pregnancy in the next year or so. I read recently that women with Type 2 diabetes have an increased risk of abnormal babies and stillbirths. Is this true?

We have known for a long time that babies of women with Type 1 diabetes had an increased risk of congenital abnormalities and of stillbirth. A lot of work has gone into trying to prevent these complications by ensuring excellent blood sugar control during the pregnancy and monitoring the baby closely to determine the optimum time for delivery. In the past it was unusual for women to develop Type 2 diabetes before the age of 40 and so pregnancy was not common in this group. We are now seeing Type 2 diabetes in a much younger age group, including school children, and it is no longer unusual for women with Type 2 diabetes to become pregnant. A recent audit of pregnancy in England, Wales and Northern Ireland (CEMACH, see the introduction to this chapter) has found that the risks to the babies of women with Type 2 diabetes are exactly the same as those for Type 1. It is therefore just as important for women with Type 2 diabetes to make sure that their diabetes is very well controlled before they conceive.

You should discuss your plans for a pregnancy with your doctor as it may be necessary to change your diabetes treatment from tablets to insulin before you become pregnant. You will need to ensure that your diabetes is very well controlled and if you are taking any tablets for blood pressure or cholesterol these will need to be stopped. Provided good control is achieved there is no reason why you should not have a successful pregnancy.

I have diabetes and would like a pregnancy soon. I have heard that women who are planning a pregnancy should take tablets called folic acid. What are these for and should I take them?

Folic acid is a naturally occurring vitamin which is present in many foods. There is good evidence that if women take extra folic acid in the early stages of pregnancy, the risk of abnormalities of the nervous system, such as spina bifida, are reduced. For women without diabetes the recommended dose is 400 μg, but women with diabetes, who are at higher risk of having a baby with an abnormality, are advised to take the higher dose of 5 mg. Your doctor will be able to prescribe this for you.

PREGNANCY MANAGEMENT

When I was seven months pregnant, I developed diabetes.
I had 8 units of insulin a day. After my baby was born,
the tests were normal and I stopped taking insulin. I would
now like another baby. My GP says I could develop
permanent diabetes but another doctor has told me that
this is very unlikely – please could you advise me?

You have had gestational diabetes (diabetes developing during pregnancy). This usually goes away when the pregnancy ends but it is very likely that diabetes will occur again in any future pregnancy. It is possible that diabetes may persist after a subsequent pregnancy, leaving you with permanent diabetes. Even if you do not have any further pregnancies, you are at high risk (greater than 1 in 2) of developing Type 2 diabetes in the future. This is because although your pancreas can produce enough insulin to cope with everyday life, its reserves are low. The extra demands of pregnancy are more than it can manage, hence the need for insulin injections and the increased risk of running out of insulin in the future. If you want to avoid diabetes in later life, you should pay particular attention to your diet and fitness, and keep your weight down to the ideal weight for your height.

Is it all right for me to breastfeed my baby if my blood
glucose is too high?

All women are encouraged to breastfeed as breast milk provides their babies with the best possible nutrition and protection against infection. There is no reason why diabetes should prevent you from breastfeeding and your baby will not be harmed in any way if your blood glucose is high. However, persistently high sugar levels may cause you to become dehydrated, which can reduce milk production. For the best results with breastfeeding, keep up a high fluid intake and try to keep a check on your blood glucose to make sure it is neither very high nor very low. It is probably best to relax your diabetes control a little to make sure that you avoid hypos as it can be very difficult to cope with a new baby if you are constantly hypo.

Breastfeeding takes a lot of energy in terms of nutritional requirements, so try to make sure that you eat regular amounts of carbohydrate. You will probably find that you need to increase your calorie intake and take less than your usual pre-pregnancy dose of insulin. Do not try to breastfeed while having a hypo: feed yourself first, so that you can feed and look after your baby safely. Always seek medical advice if you are in any doubt. If you find breastfeeding too difficult, it is perfectly all right to bottle-feed.

I am married to a man who takes insulin to control his diabetes. I have just become pregnant, so what special things do I need to do during pregnancy to ensure that it goes smoothly and without complications?

You need take no special precautions other than those taken by all pregnant women, as the fact that your husband has diabetes does not put your pregnancy at any particular risk. It is only when the mother has diabetes that strict control and careful monitoring of blood glucose become essential.

I have been told that I must keep my blood glucose levels as low as possible during pregnancy. Please can you tell me what they should be?

Your blood glucose before meals should be 4–6 mmol/litre and you should aim to be no higher than 8 mmol/L two hours after meals. If you find that this is difficult to achieve without causing a lot of hypos you should discuss the problem with your diabetes team.

I am frightened of having hypoglycaemic attacks as I have been told I need to take insulin to control my diabetes during my pregnancy. What should I do?

All people treated with insulin should be prepared for a hypo whether or not they are pregnant (see the section *Hypos* in Chapter 3) but the emphasis on tight control during pregnancy does increase the risk of hypo. Carry some form of rapidly absorbed glucose at all times – Dextro-Energy tablets are convenient. Some people prefer to carry small (125 mL) cans of Lucozade or Coca-Cola (not Diet Coke.) Your partner should be shown how to use Glucogel® (formerly Hypostop Gel) and glucagon injections as these can reverse the hypo very rapidly. Make sure you always test your blood sugar before driving.

Will any hypoglycaemic attacks that I might have during pregnancy harm the baby?

There is no evidence to suggest that even a very low blood glucose in the mother can harm the baby.

I do not have diabetes but during my last pregnancy I had what was called gestational diabetes and needed to take insulin for a few weeks. The diabetes went away after my daughter was born but I am now thinking of another pregnancy and wonder whether the same thing is likely to happen again.

You are right to think that gestational diabetes might return in your next pregnancy. During the second half of pregnancy, the body becomes resistant to insulin and larger amounts of insulin are needed to keep the blood glucose normal. Some people are unable to produce the additional insulin required and this is more likely to happen if you have a family history of diabetes, come from an ethnic group where diabetes is more common, e.g. African-Caribbean or Asian, or if you are very overweight. Many women with gestational diabetes can keep their blood sugar normal by keeping to a sugar-free diet, but some need a tablet called metformin and others require insulin. If the sugar levels are allowed to run high, the baby is likely to become fat and may have a low blood sugar for a day or two after birth. The diabetes usually goes away at the end of the pregnancy but you will be at greater risk of developing type 2 diabetes in the future. You can reduce this risk by keeping your weight as normal as possible and leading a healthy lifestyle.

COMPLICATIONS

I have had diabetes for five years. My second son was born with multiple defects and later died. Are women with diabetes more likely to have an abnormal baby?

It is a terrible tragedy to lose a baby as a result of birth defects and we hope you can pick yourself up and approach your diabetes in a positive way. The secret to a successful pregnancy is excellent blood glucose control starting before conception and continuing throughout pregnancy. There is good scientific evidence to suggest that developmental defects are caused by poor control in the first few weeks of pregnancy and that the risk of this can be reduced by ensuring perfect control when the baby is conceived. This means aiming for an HbA_{1c} of less than 7.5%. The risk of multiple congenital defects is confined to the early stages of the pregnancy. This is hardly surprising because this is the stage when the various components of the baby's body are beginning to develop and when other illnesses such as German measles (rubella) can also affect development. However, this means that there is no time to improve control once you discover that you are pregnant and it is crucial to plan the pregnancy and make sure that you have good control before you conceive. Some people have difficulty in achieving this degree of control, however hard they try. It is important to understand that the risks to the baby increase as the HbA_{1c} rises and that the closer you get to 7.5% the lower the risk.

All women planning a pregnancy are advised to take supplements of folic acid (a type of vitamin) which reduces the risk of spina bifida. The dose of folic acid recommended for women with diabetes is larger than that advised for those without diabetes. You need to start taking 5 mg of folic acid daily before you try to conceive and your doctor will be able to prescribe this for you.

Good control is also needed for the rest of the pregnancy because the development and growth of the baby can be disturbed by poor control. In particular, the baby grows faster than normal and is large in size. If the baby has to be delivered early because it is big, it will be premature and therefore at risk of the many problems that can affect premature babies.

I have read that mothers with diabetes are more likely to have babies with congenital malformations. I am thinking of a pregnancy but am terrified of having a child with an abnormality. What can I do to prevent this?

It is true that there is an association between diabetes in the mother and congenital abnormalities in her baby. We know that the most important factor influencing this is the control of the diabetes. If the HbA_{1c} is less than 7.5% at conception, the risk of congenital abnormalities is similar to that of mothers without diabetes. The higher the HbA_{1c}, the greater the risk to the development of the baby. Therefore the best thing for you to do is to make sure that your diabetes is well controlled before you conceive.

Some women with diabetes take regular medication to protect them from kidney and heart disease. These drugs can cause damage to the baby and should be stopped before you conceive. If you are uncertain about your medication you should discuss this with your doctor.

There is good evidence that taking folic acid supplements before conception protects against abnormalities such as spina bifida and in people with diabetes the higher dose of 5 mg is recommended. Your doctor will prescribe this for you.

All pregnant women are offered a blood test known as the triple test to screen for abnormalities such as Down's syndrome and spina bifida. This is carried out at 16 weeks and if abnormal, further tests will be offered to identify the problem. If these confirm an abnormality, your doctors will discuss the implications with you, and you may decide to have a termination.

Women with diabetes are also offered an abnormality scan at 20 weeks and this may be followed up with a detailed cardiac scan to identify any heart problems. If an abnormality is detected this will be discussed with you and a termination may be offered.

I have read that the babies of mothers with diabetes tend to be fat and have lung trouble shortly after birth and also there is a risk of hypoglycaemia. Is this true, and if so why does it happen?

We know that if the mother runs a high blood glucose during pregnancy, glucose crosses the placenta into the baby's circulation and causes the baby to become fat. This is because the baby's pancreas produces insulin even though the mother's cannot and the insulin converts the glucose into fat. As a result, the baby grows bigger during pregnancy and delivery has to be carried out early to avoid a difficult labour. If the mother is induced very early, there is a risk that she will not be ready to go into labour and the induction will fail, making a Caesarean section necessary. One of the complications of early delivery is that the baby's lungs may not be fully matured and this can lead to a condition known as respiratory distress syndrome (RDS). Babies with this condition need to be treated on a ventilator in the Special Care Baby Unit until their lungs are mature enough to cope.

If an early delivery is planned, most units give the mother a steroid injection prior to delivery. This helps to mature the baby's lungs and reduces the risk of RDS. The downside is that the steroids put up the blood glucose level and extra insulin will be needed for a couple of days until the effect of the steroids wears off.

If the mother's blood glucose levels are kept strictly within normal limits during pregnancy, babies are less likely to grow faster than normal and pregnancy can continue until the normal full term of 40 weeks. This avoids the risk of Caesarean section in the majority of women and RDS is rarely seen because the babies are fully mature.

Low blood glucose (hypoglycaemia) during the first few hours after birth occurs because the baby's pancreas has been producing excess amounts of insulin during the pregnancy to cover the high blood glucose levels which cross the placenta from the mother. If the mother's blood glucose is strictly controlled during pregnancy and delivery, hypoglycaemia in the baby is much less of a problem. It is normal practice to check the baby's blood sugar level when it is born and over the next 24 hours so that treatment can be given if the baby's sugar is low.

My baby was born with jaundice. Are babies of mothers with diabetes more likely to have this?

Yes, babies born to mothers with diabetes are more likely to be jaundiced. This is partly because they tend to be born early, but sometimes a full-term baby can become jaundiced. The reason for this is not clear but the problem is usually mild and if necessary the jaundice can be cleared with treatment.

I developed toxaemia during my last pregnancy and had to spend several weeks in hospital even though control of my diabetes was immaculate. Luckily everything turned out all right and I now have a beautiful healthy son. Was the toxaemia related to me having diabetes? Is it likely to recur in future pregnancies?

Women with diabetes are more prone to toxaemia (pre-eclampsia). You are not more likely to develop toxaemia in your future pregnancies – indeed the risk is lower than in your first pregnancy.

During my last pregnancy I had 'hydramnios' and my
obstetrician said that this was because I had diabetes.
Is this true? And is there anything that I can do to avoid it
happening in any future pregnancies?

Hydramnios is an excessive amount of fluid surrounding the baby and it is more common in mothers with diabetes. It is related to how strictly you control your diabetes throughout pregnancy. Our advice is that you can reduce the risk to an absolute minimum in future pregnancies by aiming to keep your HbA_{1c} and blood glucose levels as close to normal as possible from the beginning of pregnancy.

During the recent delivery of my fourth child (which went
very smoothly) I had an insulin pump into a vein during
labour. I had not had this in my previous three pregnancies,
despite having diabetes. Why did I need the pump this time?

We now know that it is very important to keep your blood glucose within normal limits during labour to minimise the risk of your baby developing a low blood glucose (hypoglycaemia) in the first few hours after birth. This is most effectively and easily done using an intravenous insulin infusion combined with some glucose given as an intravenous drip. Using this method, your blood glucose can be kept strictly regulated at the normal level until your baby has been delivered. It also ensures that if any complications arise, an anaesthetic can be given without further preparation.

My first child was delivered by Caesarean section. Do I have
to have a Caesarean section with my next pregnancy?

It depends why you had the Caesarean section. If it was performed for an obstetric reason that is likely to be present in the next pregnancy, the answer is yes. If it was performed because the first baby was large or just because you have diabetes, the answer could be no.

Some doctors do consider it safer to deliver a woman by Caesarean section if she has had a Caesarean section before. Others would allow you a 'trial of labour'. In other words, you would start labour and, if everything was satisfactory, you would be able to deliver your baby in the normal way.

My doctor tells me that I will have to have a Caesarean section because my baby is in a bad position and a little large. What sort of anaesthetic is best?

Nowadays approximately 50% of women who need a Caesarean section have an epidural rather than a general anaesthetic. If you have an epidural your legs and abdomen are made completely numb by injecting local anaesthetic solution through a needle into your lower back. You remain awake for the birth of your baby and therefore remember this major life event. In most cases an epidural is preferred because your baby receives none of the anaesthetic and therefore is not sleepy.

If you are interested in having your baby this way, you should discuss it with your obstetrician.

My baby had difficulty with breathing in his first few days in the Special Care Baby Unit. They said this was because my control of my diabetes was poor – why was this?

It sounds as if your baby had what is called respiratory distress syndrome (RDS) which occurs most commonly in premature babies and was discussed in an earlier question. It occurs in babies of mothers with diabetes where the baby has grown too quickly because of the mother's poor blood glucose control, and requires a premature delivery. It used to be a serious threat to the babies of mothers with diabetes but now it is much less common. This is because of advances in neonatal care and better control of diabetes in pregnancy resulting in fewer premature deliveries.

If there is a possibility that your baby may be born prematurely, treatment with a steroid injection can help your baby's lungs to mature. Unfortunately the steroids can upset diabetes control for about 48 hours and you will need to be in hospital for close supervision at this time.

8 | Long-term complications

Before insulin was discovered, people with diabetes did not survive long enough to develop diabetic complications as we know them today. In the early days after the great discovery in 1922, it was widely believed that insulin cured diabetes. We are now in a better position to realise that, although insulin produced nothing short of miraculous recovery in those on the verge of death, returning them to a full and active life, it does not cure the condition. Nevertheless, if insulin is used properly to achieve good diabetes control, it is possible to have a long and healthy life.

Life expectancy has increased progressively since insulin was first introduced and there are now many thousands of people who have successfully completed more than 50 years of insulin treatment. Increased longevity has brought with it a number of the so-called 'long-term complications'. Some of these complications also occur in older people who do not have diabetes. For example heart disease, stroke and poor circulation in the legs are complications which can occur as part of the ageing process. Others are not seen in people without diabetes and these are therefore the complications specific to diabetes. The three most important are eye damage (retinopathy), nerve damage (neuropathy) and kidney damage (nephropathy).

Diabetic retinopathy can lead to loss of vision and is the most common cause of blindness registration in people under 65 in the UK. Fortunately only a small proportion of people suffer complete visual loss. Diabetic neuropathy, by leading to loss of feeling, particularly in the feet, makes people susceptible to infections and occasionally gangrene, leading to the risk of amputation. It can also cause impotence. Diabetic nephropathy can cause kidney failure and is now the most common reason for referral for renal dialysis and transplantation in young people, although the numbers are very small.

It is not surprising that people dread the thought of diabetic complications. In the past they worried but did not ask about them as they were a taboo subject. Nowadays most people expect to be fully informed about the possible risk that they face and what they can do to reduce it.

There is a great deal of misinformation circulating about diabetic complications and it is important that people receive a balanced and accurate picture.

Although medical science has made impressive progress since the discovery of insulin, there is still a long way to go. There is overwhelming scientific evidence to show that the risk of complications is directly related to blood glucose control. Thus, prevention of complications is possible by tight control of the blood glucose concentration. The evidence comes from a very large clinical trial carried out in this country: the UK Prospective Diabetes Study (UKPDS), which provided indisputable evidence that complications can be avoided by strict blood glucose control, aiming for an HbA_{1c} of 7%. There is more information about the trial in the introduction to Chapter 4: **Monitoring and control.**

Some of the questions in this chapter relating to eyes and feet are not strictly questions about complications, but as they do not easily fit in anywhere else in the book they have been included in this chapter under their specific headings.

GENERAL QUESTIONS

Can someone with diabetes controlled only by diet suffer from diabetic complications?

Complications may occur with any type of diabetes. The cause of diabetic complications is not completely understood. Unquestionably the main cause of long-term complications is poor blood glucose control over a number of years but this is not the whole story and some people with prolonged poor control do not run into any problems. Presumably people like this are protected in some way – possibly by genetic factors. The duration of diabetes (the length of time for which you have had it, whether diagnosed or not) is also important: complications are rare in the first few years and occur more commonly after many years. The longer the duration, the higher the risk.

People treated with diet alone are usually diagnosed in middle or later life. At the time of diagnosis, the disease may have been present for a long time, often many years, without the person being aware of it, and therefore without any attempt being made to control it. Thus it is not surprising that complications can occur in some people even when they are treated with diet alone. Good control in these people is clearly just as important as in people who have treatment with tablets or who have Type 1 diabetes.

What are the complications and what should I keep a lookout for to ensure that they are picked up as soon as possible?

The complications specific to diabetes are known as diabetic retinopathy, neuropathy and nephropathy.

- Retinopathy means damage to the retina at the back of the eye.

- Neuropathy means damage to the nerves. This can affect nerves supplying any part of the body but is generally referred to as either 'peripheral' when affecting nerves supplying muscles and skin, or as 'autonomic' when affecting nerves supplying organs such as the bladder, the bowel and the heart.

- Nephropathy is damage affecting the kidneys, which in the first instance makes them more leaky, so that albumin (protein) appears in the urine. At a later stage it may affect the function of the kidneys and in severe cases lead to kidney failure.

The best way of detecting complications early is to visit your doctor or clinic for regular review. You should have a check once a year, either at your doctor's surgery or at the hospital clinic so that complications can be detected at an early stage. Most areas now offer annual retinal photography to screen for diabetic eye changes. It is important to make use of this service.

Prevention is, however, clearly better than treatment and, if you can control your diabetes well you will be less likely to suffer these complications.

I am very worried that I might develop complications after some years of having diabetes. Is it possible to avoid complications in later life? If so, how?

We believe that all people could avoid complications if they were able to control their diabetes from the day that they were diagnosed. There are now many cases on record of people who have had Type 1 diabetes for 50 years or more and are completely free from any signs of complications. Things are a bit different for Type 2 diabetes, which may be present for many years without causing any symptoms. Some people may be unfortunate enough to develop a complication, such as a foot ulcer, before diabetes itself is diagnosed.

The best advice we can give you on how to avoid complications is to take the control of your blood glucose and diabetes seriously from the outset and to attend regularly for review and supervision by somebody experienced in the management of people with diabetes. Focus on learning how to look after yourself in such a way that you can achieve and maintain a normal HbA$_{1c}$ level (see the section *Haemoglobin A$_{1c}$* in Chapter 4). If you can do that and keep your HbA$_{1c}$ normal, you can look forward to a life free from the risk of diabetic complications.

To what extent are the complications of diabetes genetically determined?

This is a very difficult question to answer. Most specialists believe that there is a hereditary factor which predisposes some people to develop certain complications and makes others relatively immune from them. So far, scientific evidence for this is not very strong but there is a lot of work in progress in this field at the moment.

I have recently been told I have Type 2 diabetes and have read that this may reduce my life span. Is this true?

Any effect diabetes may have on life span depends on the age at which diabetes is diagnosed. The older you are at diagnosis, the closer your expected life span is to someone who does not have diabetes. The biggest threat to people with Type 2 diabetes is the increased risk of heart attack and stroke. Fortunately, great strides have been made over the last few years in reducing these risks and most people with Type 2 diabetes find that their doctor advises them to take a cholesterol-lowering tablet called a statin, along with a very low dose of aspirin. A number of studies have shown that by taking these tablets the risk of heart attack and stroke is reduced by about 25%. If you have high blood pressure, it is very important to take treatment to bring this down and some people need a combination of three or four drugs to achieve the target blood pressure of less than 140/80. It may come as a shock to find that once you have diabetes you suddenly need to take a large number of tablets – you may need tablets for your diabetes as well – but there is no doubt

that by controlling your blood glucose, blood pressure and cholesterol you can increase your life expectancy. Cigarette smoking greatly
increases the risk of heart attack and stroke for people with diabetes
and if you are a smoker you should do your best to stop.

*My diabetes specialist has said that it does not follow that
badly controlled people get all the side effects and ill health
in later life and the reverse may often be true. Is this
really so?*

There is an element of truth in this but the word 'often' should be
replaced by 'very occasionally'. Well controlled people are much
less likely to become ill and develop side effects, whereas people who
have unstable and unbalanced diabetes frequently develop ill health
and side effects in later life. This has been confirmed by the results of
the UK Prospective Diabetes Study (UKPDS) – there is more information about this trial in the section *Why monitor?* in Chapter 4.

*For the last two years my cheeks have become increasingly
hollow although my weight is static – is this due to diabetes?*

Quite a lot of middle-aged and elderly people become slim up
top and pear shaped below, whether or not they have diabetes.
However, there is a rare form of diabetes called lipoatrophic diabetes
and this could possibly be the explanation for the hollowing of your
cheeks. This is not a complication of diabetes but a rare form of the
condition. Mention it to your doctor the next time you go for a review.

EYES

I had a tendency towards short-sightedness before being diagnosed as having diabetes. Is this likely to increase my chances of developing eye complications later on?

Short-sightedness does not make the slightest difference to the risk of developing diabetic eye complications – in fact it has been said that those with severe short-sightedness may actually be less, rather than more, prone to retinopathy.

Vision may vary with changes in diabetes control. Large fluctuations in blood glucose levels can temporarily alter the shape of the lens in the eye and this alters its focusing capacity. It is not uncommon for people with consistently high blood glucose levels to have difficulty with distance vision. Once diabetes is controlled and the blood glucose returns to more normal levels, vision changes again, sometimes causing difficulty with near vision and therefore with reading.

These changes in vision are most likely to occur at the time diabetes is diagnosed and can be frightening, if the reason is not understood. After three or four weeks of good diabetic control, vision always returns to the prediabetes state. We always advise people with newly-diagnosed diabetes not to change their glasses until their blood sugar has been stable for about four weeks.

As someone with diabetes, I know I should have my eyes checked, but how often should this be?

Once a year should be enough if your diabetes is well controlled, your vision normal and you have no signs of complications. Diabetes can cause changes at the back of the eye (retinopathy). In the early stages, these changes do not affect vision but it is important to detect them as soon as possible so that treatment can be given to keep your vision normal. Nowadays, screening for retinopathy is usually carried out by digital photography and the Diabetes NSF states that this should be available to every person with diabetes.

> *I have just been discovered to have diabetes and the glasses that I have had for several years seem no longer suitable, but my doctor tells me not to get them changed until my diabetes has been brought under control – is this right?*

Yes. When the glucose concentration in the body rises, this affects the focusing ability of the eyes, but it is only a temporary effect, and your vision will return to normal once the glucose has been brought under control. If you change your glasses now you will be able to see better for a short time but as soon as your diabetes is brought under control you will need to change them again. It is better to follow your doctor's advice and wait until your diabetes has been controlled for at least a month before going back to the optician.

> *Who is the best person to check my eyes once a year?*

In the past, eye checks have been done in various ways but the Diabetes NSF recommends that every person with diabetes should be offered an annual eye check in the form of digital retinal photography (see next question on eye photography).

> *I have been sent an appointment for eye photographs. What will this involve?*

There are two parts to the examination. The first is to test visual acuity, which measures your ability to read the letters on a chart. The second is to have the back of your eyes photographed. You will need drops in your eyes beforehand to enlarge the pupils in order to obtain good quality photographs. The drops may cause blurred vision for up to three hours afterwards and you should not drive until your vision has returned to normal. If it is a very bright day, you may suffer from glare while your pupils are dilated and sunglasses will prevent this. Each eye will be photographed once or twice using a flash camera. You may see some bright colours for a few seconds after the flash but these will go very quickly. If abnormalities are seen on the photographs, you will be referred to an eye specialist.

Last time I was having my eyes checked from the chart, the nurse made me look through a small pinhole. Why was this?

The pinhole acts as a universal correcting lens. If your vision improves when looking through the pinhole, it suggests that you may be helped by spectacles.

Why does diabetes affect the eyes?

A simple question but one that is difficult to answer. Current research indicates strongly that it is the excess glucose in the bloodstream that directly damages the eyes, mainly by affecting the lining of the small blood vessels that carry blood to the retina. The damage to these vessels seems to be directly related to how high the blood glucose is and how long it has been raised.

I have had diabetes for 20 years and seem to be quite well. Following my last eye photograph, I had a letter to say that I had some mild diabetic changes and would be referred to an eye specialist. Am I about to go blind?

There is no need for alarm. It would be surprising if there were no changes in your eyes after 20 years of diabetes. It is important that you see an eye specialist at an early stage so that if treatment is required, it can be given before your vision is affected.

I have been diagnosed with retinopathy. Can you explain more about this?

Retinopathy is a condition affecting the back of the eye (the retina). It may occur in people with long-standing diabetes, particularly those in whom control has not been very good. There is a gradual change in the blood vessels (arteries and veins) at the back of the eye which can lead to deterioration in vision. This may be due either to deposits in a vital area at the back of the eye or to bleeding into the eye from abnormal blood vessels.

Retinopathy may be diagnosed by examination of the eye with an ophthalmoscope or by retinal photography. It can usually be detected long before it leads to any disturbance in vision. Laser treatment at this stage usually stops further deterioration.

On a recent TV programme it was stated that people with diabetes over 40 years of age were likely to become blind. This has shocked me and my partner who is 46 years old and has had Type 2 diabetes for ten years. Is it really true?

Many adults who have had diabetes for ten years will have some changes in the eyes (retinopathy). However, these are usually very minor and do not affect vision. Only a very small proportion of people actually go blind, probably no more than 7% of those who have had diabetes for 30 years or more. This figure is likely to reduce further over the next few years because the national retinopathy screening progamme has been set up to detect retinopathy at an early stage, when treatment can prevent damage to vision. We have known for 30 years that laser treatment is effective in treating diabetic retin-opathy but sadly, some people do not realise they have a problem with their eyes until irreversible damage has been done. The retinal screening programme offers annual retinal photographs to everyone with diabetes. Your partner should be offered an appointment. If he is not, he should ask his GP or practice nurse about the local arrange-ments for retinal screening. It is important to understand that people with well controlled diabetes are much less likely to develop retinopathy than those with poor control.

Can I wear contact lenses and if so would you recommend hard or soft ones?

The fact that you have diabetes should not interfere with your use of contact lenses or influence the sort of lens that you are given. The best person to advise you would be an ophthalmologist or qualified optician specialising in prescribing and fitting contact lenses. It would be sensible to let him or her know that you have diabetes and you must follow the advice given, particularly to prevent infection – but this applies to everyone, with or without diabetes.

I get flashes of light and specks across my vision. Are they symptoms of serious eye trouble?

Although people with diabetes do get eye trouble, this does not normally cause flashing lights or specks across the vision. You should discuss it with your own doctor who will want to examine your eyes in case there is any problem.

My father has diabetes and was recently told he had cataracts. Is this connected with his diabetes?

Cataracts occur in older people whether or not they have diabetes. However, they tend to occur at an earlier age in people with diabetes. The ageing process affects the substance that makes up the lens of the eye causing it to wrinkle and become less transparent than normal. Eventually it becomes so opaque that it becomes difficult to see properly through it. Your father's doctor should arrange for him to see an eye specialist.

The last time I was tested at the clinic, I was told that I had developed microaneurysms. What on earth are these?

Microaneurysms are little balloon-like swellings or dilatations in the very small blood vessels (capillaries) supplying the retina at the back of the eye. They are one of the earliest signs that the high blood glucose levels seen in poorly controlled diabetes have damaged the lining to these capillaries. They do not interfere with vision, but give an early warning that retinopathy has begun to develop. There is evidence to show that these can get better with the introduction of perfect control (target HbA_{1c} less than 7.5%) whereas, at later stages of diabetic retinopathy, reversal is not usually possible. Anyone who has microaneurysms must have regular eye checks, so that any serious developments are detected at an early stage. You have been picked up early so now is the time to make sure that your glucose control is impeccable!

I shall be going to have laser treatment soon on my eyes. What will this involve?

Laser treatment uses a narrow beam of intense light to cause very small burns on the retina at the back of the eye. It is used in the treatment of many eye conditions including diabetic retinopathy. The laser is directed at parts of the retina not used for detailed vision, sparing the important areas required for reading, etc. This form of treatment arrests or delays the progress of retinopathy, provided that it is given in adequate amounts at an early stage before useful vision is lost. It is sometimes necessary to give small doses of laser treatment intermittently over many years, although occasionally it can all be dealt with over a relatively short period. Although this treatment sounds quite alarming, it is not usually painful though it may cause minor discomfort.

My doctor used the term 'photocoagulation' the other day. Is this the same as laser treatment? Will it damage my eyes at all?

Photocoagulation is indeed treatment of retinopathy by lasers. It is uncommon for the treatment to damage the eyes, but strictly speaking it is possible. Occasionally the scar produced by photocoagulation can spread and involve vital parts of the retina so that vision is affected. The vast majority of people who have laser therapy do not notice any change in their vision. People who need repeated laser treatment may notice that their night vision is poor or that their field of vision is reduced. Photocoagulation can also very rarely result in rupture of a blood vessel, which causes bleeding. After a great deal of photocoagulation there is a slight risk of damage to the lens causing a type of cataract. Although this may sound rather worrying, there is very strong evidence to show that if you have serious retinopathy, laser treatment is the best way to preserve vision and the risk of damage as a result of the laser treatment is far less than the risk to your sight if the retinopathy is left untreated. It is important to realise that laser treatment cannot reverse any damage that has already occurred but it can prevent further deterioration.

I have glaucoma. Is this related to diabetes?

Possibly. Although glaucoma can occur quite commonly in people who do not have diabetes, there is a slightly increased risk in those who do. This is usually confined to those who have advanced diabetic eye problems (proliferative retinopathy).

Very occasionally the eye drops used to enlarge the pupil can precipitate an attack of glaucoma (increased pressure inside the eye). The signs of this are pain in the affected eye together with blurring of vision which may come on some hours after the drops have been put in. Should this occur you must seek urgent medical advice either from your own doctor or from the accident and emergency department of your local hospital. It is reversible with rapid treatment but can cause serious damage if ignored.

Every time I receive my copy of Balance, Diabetes UK's magazine, I have the impression that the print gets smaller. Is this true or is there something wrong with my eyes?

Eyesight tends to deteriorate with age, whether or not someone has diabetes. First you should visit your optician and have your eyesight checked to see whether it can be improved with glasses, as this may be all that is required. You should mention the fact that you have diabetes to your optician.

My eyesight has become very poor and my optician says it cannot be improved. I have increasing difficulty in reading. Is there any help available?

For people with eye problems severe enough to prevent reading, there are ways of helping. *Balance*, for example, is available to members of Diabetes UK as a cassette recording and this service is free of charge although, to satisfy Post Office regulations, you have to have a certificate of blindness before the cassette can be sent to you.

Public libraries can also help – most carry a wide selection of books in large type and also lend books on cassette and CD. Some larger libraries now have Kurtzweil machines, which can translate printed material into speech so that, in effect, they can read to you, although the 'voice' sounds a bit mechanical. This can be useful for any confidential material that you might not want another person to read to you. Libraries usually have these machines in rooms on their own so, once you have been shown how to use them, you can be quite private.

The Royal National Institute of the Blind also has an excellent talking book service. *Diabetes: Answers at your fingertips* is available as a talking book from the RNIB.

FEET, PODIATRY AND FOOTWEAR

I have just developed diabetes and have been warned that I am much more likely to get into trouble with my feet and need to take great care of them – what does this mean?

Diabetes can damage the nerves in the feet, reducing sensation and increasing the risk of injury and ulceration. If you keep your diabetes well controlled, have no loss of sensation and good circulation to your feet, you are no more at risk than a person without diabetes. If you do have nerve damage or poor circulation, you must protect your feet by taking the following precautions:

- inspecting your feet daily;
- keeping your toenails properly trimmed;
- avoiding badly fitting shoes.

When you have diabetes you should have access to the local registered podiatrist, who will check your feet and advise you, free of charge, on any questions that you may have.

As someone with diabetes, do I have to take any special precautions when cutting my toenails?

It is important for everyone to cut their toenails to follow the shape of the end of the toe, and not cut deep into the corners. Your toenails should not be cut too short, and you should not use any sharp instrument to clean down the sides of the nails. All this is to avoid the possibility of ingrowing toenails. If you have problems cutting your toenails consult your registered podiatrist.

I have had diabetes for ten years and as far as I can see it is quite under control and I am told that I am free from complications, but I cannot help worrying about the possibility of developing gangrene in the feet – can you tell me what it is and what causes it?

G angrene results from tissue death. It can occur in any part of the body but most commonly affects the toes and fingers. Gangrene can occur in anyone with poor circulation and people with diabetes develop it only if they have a serious lack of blood supply to their feet. It can also be caused by smoking, which is the main cause of clogged-up blood vessels and the combination of smoking and diabetes more than doubles the risk of gangrene.

There is another form of gangrene, which is caused by infection and is more common in people with diabetes. This usually affects the feet of people who have reduced sensation because of diabetic neuropathy (see the introduction to this chapter) and can occur even in the presence of a good blood supply. Any infected break in the skin of your feet must be taken seriously and treated promptly. If you are worried about anything to do with your feet, you should consult your doctor or podiatrist immediately. If the infection persists, ask to be referred to your local Diabetic Foot Team.

I have a thick callus on the top of one of my toes – can I use a corn plaster on this?

N o, do not use any corn remedies on your feet. They often contain an acid which softens the skin and increases the risk of an infection. Consult a registered podiatrist to have it treated. Contacts can be found on the websites for the Society of Chiropodists and Podiatrists and the Health Professions Council. As you have diabetes you should have access to a registered podiatrist who will treat you free of charge.

I have diabetes treated with insulin and have developed
athlete's foot. Do I have to take any special precautions about
using the powder and cream given to me by my doctor?

No. Athlete's foot is very common and is due to a fungal infection, which should respond quickly to treatment with the appropriate antifungal preparation; this can be bought without prescription. Do not forget the usual precautions of keeping your feet clean, drying them carefully and changing socks daily. Try not to wear the same footwear every day.

Will I get bunions because I have diabetes?

No. Bunions are no more common in people who have diabetes than in those who do not.

I have had diabetes for 25 years and I have been warned that
the sensation in my feet is not normal. I am troubled with
an ingrowing toenail on my big toe, which often gets red but
does not hurt – what should I do?

You should urgently seek help and advice in case it is infected. If so, you are at risk of the infection spreading without you being aware of it, because it would hurt less than in someone with normal sensation. This is potentially a serious situation, so see your doctor or podiatrist straight away.

I am 67 and have had diabetes for 15 years. As far as I can
tell my feet are quite healthy but, as my vision is not very
good, I find it difficult to inspect my feet properly – what can
I do about it?

Do you have a friend or relative who could look at your feet regularly and trim your nails? If this is not possible, then the sensible thing to do would be to see a podiatrist regularly. Ask your

GP or diabetes clinic about local arrangements for seeing a registered podiatrist.

Do I have to pay for chiropody?

Most hospital diabetes departments provide a chiropody (podiatry) service free of charge. Outside the hospital service, podiatry under the NHS is based on locally agreed priority groups. Most districts consider people with diabetes as a priority group and do offer free podiatry. You should check locally before obtaining treatment. If you are seeing a podiatrist privately, make sure that he or she is registered (see question on corn plasters, above, for details).

How can I tell whether diabetes is affecting my feet?

Diabetes may affect the feet in two major ways. The first is caused by reduced blood supply from arterial thickening, sometimes called 'hardening of the arteries' or atherosclerosis. This leads to poor circulation with cold feet, even in warm weather, and cramps in the calf when you are walking (intermittent claudication). Poor circulation is not confined to people with diabetes and becomes increasingly common with age, particularly in people who smoke. The combination of diabetes and smoking is particularly harmful and in severe cases this can progress to gangrene.

The second way that diabetes can affect the feet is through damage to the nerves (neuropathy), which reduces the feeling of pain and awareness of extremes of temperature. When your feet are insensitive, it is easy to damage them without realising it, for example by wearing poorly fitting footwear. Neuropathy can be quite difficult to detect unless the feet are examined by an expert. Once a year, one of the health professionals helping you to manage your diabetes should examine your feet for signs of reduced blood supply or nerve damage. They should tell you if there is evidence that diabetes is affecting your feet.

The danger is that any minor damage to the foot, whether from a cut or abrasion or a badly fitting shoe, will not cause the usual painful reaction, so that damage can result from continued injury or from infection. It is important that you know whether the sensation in your feet is normal or reduced. Make sure that you ask your doctor or nurse about this at your next review.

I have just found out I have diabetes and have been told not to walk barefoot. Why is this?

It is well known that people with diabetes are prone to problems with their feet which, for the most part, can be avoided. Once diabetes has been present for a few years, it may reduce sensation in the feet, making them more susceptible to damage. Sometimes the loss of sensation comes on so gradually that the person is not aware that they have this potentially serious problem. Walking barefoot carries a risk of minor injury, which can turn into something much worse if the normal warning signs are missing. People who have lost sensation in their feet are especially at risk at holiday times when they may walk longer distances or even burn their feet on hot sand.

What special care should I take of my feet during the winter?

In older people with diabetes, the blood supply to the feet may not be very good and this will make their feet more vulnerable to damage by severe cold. As winter is cold and wet, we tend to wear warmer clothing, and previously comfortable shoes may become unpleasantly tight when worn with thick woolly socks or stockings. This may reduce the circulation to the feet and can numb the sensation completely, leading to damage. All these effects will be made worse if your feet become wet.

Make sure your shoes are comfortable, fit well, and allow room for you to wear an adequately thick pair of socks, preferably made of wool or other absorbent material. Use weather-proof shoes, overshoes or boots if you are going to be out for any length of time in the

Feet Facts

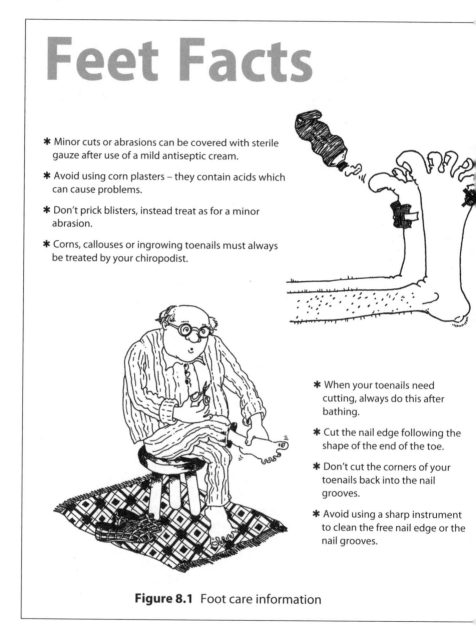

* Minor cuts or abrasions can be covered with sterile gauze after use of a mild antiseptic cream.

* Avoid using corn plasters – they contain acids which can cause problems.

* Don't prick blisters, instead treat as for a minor abrasion.

* Corns, callouses or ingrowing toenails must always be treated by your chiropodist.

* When your toenails need cutting, always do this after bathing.

* Cut the nail edge following the shape of the end of the toe.

* Don't cut the corners of your toenails back into the nail grooves.

* Avoid using a sharp instrument to clean the free nail edge or the nail grooves.

Figure 8.1 Foot care information

* If your skin is too dry, apply a small amount of emollient cream (e.g. E45).

* Check and bathe your feet every day, then pat dry gently, particularly between the toes.

* If your skin is moist, dab gently with surgical spirit and then dust lightly with talcum powder.

* Remove hot water bottles before getting into bed, and switch off your electric blanket.

* If thick woollen bed-socks are worn, they must be loose fitting.

* Be careful not to sit too close to radiators or fires.

* Choose shoes which provide good support. They must be broad, long and deep enough. Check that you can wriggle all your toes.

* Shoes should have a fastening.

* Check shoes daily for any small objects, such as hairpins, stones or buttons.

* If socks have ridges or seams, wear them inside out. Loose fitting ones are best.

* Avoid very hot baths.

* Always dry your feet carefully after bathing.

rain or snow, and dry your feet carefully if they get wet. Do not put your cold – and slightly numb – feet straight onto a hot-water bottle or near a hot fire because you may find that, when the feeling comes back, the heat is excessive and chilblains may occur. Feet also need protection during the summer as wearing open sandals can cause problems from possible damage by sharp stones, etc.

How can I give continual protection to my feet?

It is extremely difficult. If the sensation in your feet is normal, then generally you have very little need to worry but, if there is even slight numbness of your feet, you should check them daily and ask someone else to look at the areas that you have difficulty seeing. (If there is no one to ask you could try using a mirror to look at the soles of your feet.) You are looking for signs mentioned in the Foot Care Rules (Figure 8.2). If your circulation is poor, try hard to keep your feet warm and well protected.

I have suffered from foot ulcers for many years and would be grateful if you could suggest something to help my problem.

You should not attempt to treat these yourself. Seek medical advice and expert podiatry, usually provided by your local Diabetic Foot Team. Foot ulcers in people with diabetes are usually caused by reduced sensation in the feet (neuropathy) and you should have your feet examined by your specialist to find out whether this is the case. If so, you need to attend for regular podiatry and learn all the ways of avoiding trouble when sensation is reduced. You may need special shoes made by a shoe fitter (an orthotist), which your consultant or podiatrist can arrange. Another form of treatment for people with foot ulcers is to use a removeable plaster cast, such as is used to immobilise fractured bones. These can be made from a light plastic material called Scotchcast, which provides maximum protection to an ulcerated foot.

*I have so many other things to remember – can you give me
a simple list of rules for foot care?*

The Foot Care Rules (Figure 8.2) are aimed specifically at those who have either poor blood supply (ischaemia) or nerve damage (neuropathy). If you have poor eyesight then you should get somebody else with good eyesight to help you inspect and care for your feet. The rules are shown in a more entertaining form in Figure 8.1.

I have a swollen foot – is this to do with my diabetes?

Swelling of both feet, especially towards the end of the day, is not directly related to diabetes and there are a number of possible causes, some of which may benefit from treatment. The best thing would be to speak to your doctor about this.

Sometimes people with diabetes and reduced sensation in their feet (neuropathy) can develop a swollen, painful foot which is warm to the touch and can look like a sprained ankle. This uncommon condition is called a Charcot foot and it is important to recognise and treat it at an early stage. If left untreated the foot may change shape, which will put it at increased risk of ulceration in the future. The Charcot process may start as a result of a minor injury to the foot and the diagnosis is often delayed because the changes are thought to be due to a sprain. It is very important to see your GP or podiatrist as soon as possible as if you have this condition you will need specialist treatment from the Diabetes Foot Team.

The treatment for a Charcot foot is to immobilise it in a cast – this can be a traditional plaster cast or an aircast (sometimes called a 'Beckham Boot') to stop the foot changing shape. Sometimes tablets normally used for osteoporosis (bisphosphonates) are prescribed to strengthen the bones. It can take several months for a Charcot foot to stabilise but if during this time you protect your foot from changing shape, it will be worth the inconvenience.

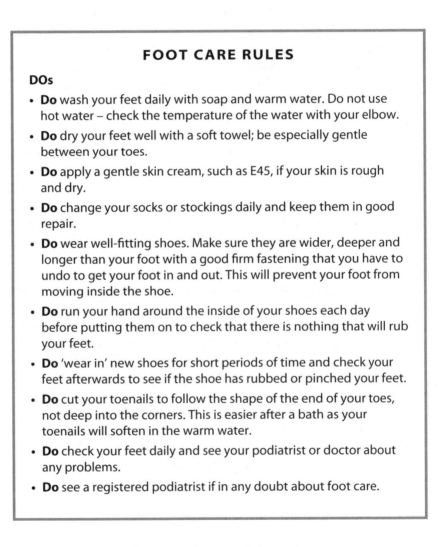

FOOT CARE RULES

DOs

- **Do** wash your feet daily with soap and warm water. Do not use hot water – check the temperature of the water with your elbow.

- **Do** dry your feet well with a soft towel; be especially gentle between your toes.

- **Do** apply a gentle skin cream, such as E45, if your skin is rough and dry.

- **Do** change your socks or stockings daily and keep them in good repair.

- **Do** wear well-fitting shoes. Make sure they are wider, deeper and longer than your foot with a good firm fastening that you have to undo to get your foot in and out. This will prevent your foot from moving inside the shoe.

- **Do** run your hand around the inside of your shoes each day before putting them on to check that there is nothing that will rub your feet.

- **Do** 'wear in' new shoes for short periods of time and check your feet afterwards to see if the shoe has rubbed or pinched your feet.

- **Do** cut your toenails to follow the shape of the end of your toes, not deep into the corners. This is easier after a bath as your toenails will soften in the warm water.

- **Do** check your feet daily and see your podiatrist or doctor about any problems.

- **Do** see a registered podiatrist if in any doubt about foot care.

Figure 8.2 Foot care information

DON'Ts

- **Do not** soak your feet.
- **Do not** put your feet on hot-water bottles or sit too close to a fire or radiator, and avoid extremes of cold and heat.
- **Do not** use corn paints or plasters or attempt to cut your own corns with knives or razors under any circumstances.
- **Do not** neglect even slight injuries to your feet.
- **Do not** walk barefoot.
- **Do not** let your feet get dry and cracked. Use E45 or hand lotion to keep the skin soft. Avoid putting moisturiser between the toes.
- **Do not** cut your toenails too short or dig down the sides of your nails.
- **Do not** smoke.

Seek advice immediately if you notice any of the following:

- Any colour change in your legs or feet.
- Any discharge from a break or crack in the skin, or from a corn or from beneath a toenail.
- Any swelling, throbbing or signs of inflammation (redness or heat) in any part of your foot.

First aid measures

- Minor injuries can be treated at home provided that professional help is sought if the injury does not improve quickly.
- Minor cuts and abrasions should be cleaned gently with cotton wool or gauze and warm salt water. A clean dressing should be lightly bandaged in place.
- If blisters occur, do not prick them. If they burst, dress as for minor cuts.
- Never use strong medicaments such as iodine.
- Never place adhesive strapping directly over a wound: always apply a dressing first

KIDNEY DAMAGE

It's bad enough having diabetes. If I'm also at risk of kidney damage, what should I look for?

Diabetes may affect the kidneys in several ways, and the routine urine and blood tests that you have once a year, either at your doctor's surgery or at your diabetes clinic, can detect changes at an early stage, when it is possible for treatment to protect against further damage.

Large amounts of glucose in the urine put you at risk of infection that can spread from the bladder (cystitis) up to the kidneys (pyelonephritis). Sometimes long-standing kidney infections may cause very few symptoms and are only revealed by routine urine tests.

People with long-standing and poorly controlled diabetes are at risk of damage to the small blood vessels supplying the kidney, in the same way that the retina of the eye may be affected. This does not produce any symptoms but will be detected with a urine test carried out by your doctor or nurse. Most clinics now test for 'micro-albuminuria', which as the name implies is a microscopic amount of albumin (protein) in the urine. This is a very useful test as it can detect very minor kidney damage, which will respond to treatment.

With more severe kidney disease, large amounts of albumin may be lost in the urine. This may make the urine froth and can lead to a build-up of fluid in the body, which in turn leads to swelling around the ankles (oedema). Over many years, these changes may progress to kidney failure. This is usually detected by blood tests and urine tests years before the symptoms develop.

I have developed kidney failure. Will it be possible to have dialysis or even a transplant although I have diabetes?

Yes. The majority of people who are unfortunate enough to get kidney failure are suitable for both forms of treatment.

Dialysis (or renal replacement therapy) is of two major types. The older type is haemodialysis where the blood is washed in a special machine three times a week. The more recent form of dialysis is known as CAPD (chronic ambulatory peritoneal dialysis) where fluid is washed in and out of the abdomen three or four times a day. The benefit of CAPD is that it can be carried out at home and does not need sophisticated machinery. People with diabetes seem to be very good at learning this method, which is simpler and cheaper than haemodialysis.

Transplantation is the aim of most dialysis programmes, but the supply of suitable kidneys is a limiting factor. The source of kidneys is either from people dying accidentally or from a family member who has agreed to give one of their kidneys to a relative with kidney failure. A normal person can manage perfectly well with one kidney without reducing their life expectancy provided the kidney does not get damaged. The donor will, of course, have to have an operation and will be slightly more vulnerable as a result because they will have only one kidney to rely on instead of two.

I was found to have protein (albumin) in my urine when I last attended the diabetes clinic – what does this mean?

If it was only a trace of protein, it may mean nothing, but you should have your urine checked again to make sure it is now clear. If the protein is still present, it suggests either that you could have an infection in the bladder or kidney (cystitis or pyelonephritis) or that you have developed a degree of diabetic kidney damage (nephropathy). There are many other causes of protein (albumin) in the urine and it may not be related to your diabetes. If the protein is always present in every urine specimen, this should be investigated, and you should ask to be kept informed of the results of the tests.

At my last clinic visit I was told that I had micro-albuminuria. What is this?

One of the effects diabetes can have on the kidney is to cause protein (albumin) to leak into the urine. At first this happens in microscopic amounts, but with time the albumin in the urine (albuminuria) increases and this can lead to fluid retention and ankle swelling. A very sensitive test has been developed to detect albumin at the microscopic stage (microalbuminuria) and your doctor or nurse should ask you to provide an early morning urine sample once a year so that you can be tested for microalbuminuria. The reason for screening for kidney damage at such an early stage is that if it is detected, microalbuminuria can be stabilised or even reversed by keeping the blood pressure absolutely normal and by treating you with a tablet known as an ACE inhibitor. For the same reason it is important to keep your diabetes as well controlled as possible.

At my last diabetes check my doctor told me that I had a condition called microalbuminuria and that I needed to take a blood pressure tablet to protect my kidneys, even though he says my blood pressure is normal. I feel very well and don't like the idea of taking tablets – is this really necessary?

It is always difficult to accept the need to take treatment when you are feeling perfectly well and most people are reluctant to take tablets in these circumstances. However, there is good evidence that microalbuminuria can be halted, and can even be reversed, by treatment with an ACE inhibitor and your doctor is giving you good advice.

NERVE DAMAGE

There are a number of conditions that can affect the nervous system of someone with diabetes: diabetic neuritis, diabetic neuropathy, autoimmune neuropathy and diabetic amyotrophy. We discuss these below.

> *I have been on insulin for three years. Eighteen months ago I started to get pains in both legs and could barely walk. Despite treatment I am still suffering. Can you tell me what can be done to ease this pain?*

There are many causes of leg pains, and only one is due specifically to diabetes. This is a particularly vicious form of nerve damage called neuritis, which causes singularly unpleasant pain, chiefly in the feet or thighs, or sometimes both. The pain is often described as pins and needles, or constant burning, and is often worse at night causing lack of sleep. Contact with clothes or bedclothes is often acutely uncomfortable.

Fortunately this form of neuritis is rather uncommon and always disappears, although it may last for many months before subsiding. Sometimes good control of your diabetes will help to alleviate the symptoms and speed recovery. Relief can be obtained by simple painkillers, but there are also some drugs which were developed for other purposes which have been shown to be effective in relieving pain due to neuropathy. The first choice is the antidepressant amitriptyline. If this fails, gabapentin or pregabalin, which were first developed for epilepsy, should be tried. Sometimes sleeping tablets can help. As a general rule, painful neuropathy improves eventually but this can take some time.

I have had diabetes for many years but my general health is good and I am very stable. During the last year, however, I have developed an extreme soreness on the soles of my feet whenever pressure has been applied, such as when digging with a spade, standing on ladders, walking on hard ground or stones, even when applying the accelerator in the car. If I thump an object with the palm of my hand, I suffer the same soreness. The pain is extreme and sometimes lasts for a day or so. Could you tell me if you have heard of this condition in other people and what is the reason for it?

These symptoms may be due to diabetic neuropathy, a condition of damage to the nerves, which sometimes occurs in long-standing diabetes. It affects the feet more often than other parts of the body and may cause painful tingling or burning sensations in the feet, although numbness is perhaps more common. Strict control of your diabetes is important for the prevention and treatment of this complication – it can be made worse by moderate or high alcohol consumption.

I have diabetes controlled on diet alone. I suffer from neuritis in my face. My GP says there is no apparent reason for this but I wondered if it had anything to do with my diabetes.

Not necessarily, as there are a number of types of neuritis that can affect the face, which have absolutely nothing to do with diabetes. Examples include both shingles (Herpes zoster) and Bell's palsy, although, of course, both these conditions can affect people with diabetes.

There are forms of diabetic neuritis that do affect the face: one form occasionally affects the muscles of the eye leading to double vision, while another form can cause numbness and tingling. There is also a very rare complication known as 'gustatory sweating' where sweating breaks out across the head and scalp at the start of a meal.

I have recently been told that the tingling sensation in my fingers is due to carpal tunnel syndrome and not neuropathy as was first thought. Can you please explain the difference?

Carpal tunnel syndrome commonly occurs in people who do not have diabetes; the wrist compresses the nerve supplying the skin over the fingers, the palm of the hand and some of the muscles in the hand. Occasionally injections of hydrocortisone or related steroids into the wrist will relieve it. Sometimes a small operation at the wrist to relieve the tension on the nerve may be required. This usually brings about a dramatic relief of any associated pain and a recovery of sensation and muscle strength with time.

Diabetic neuropathy more commonly affects the feet than the hands and is usually a painless loss of sensation starting with the tips of the toes or fingers and moving up the legs or arms. It is only occasionally painful and may be difficult to treat. It is due to generalised damage to the nerves, not to compression of any one nerve and is often described as 'glove and stocking'.

I have had diabetes for 27 years and have recently had a lot of trouble with diarrhoea. My doctor says it may be caused by diabetes. Could you explain why this should happen now and how it can be treated?

Diabetic diarrhoea is one of a number of problems which can be caused by autonomic neuropathy. This occurs when there is damage to the nerves supplying the 'automatic' bodily functions such as bowels, bladder and stomach. It is an uncommon condition, which can develop after many years of diabetes. For reasons which are not well understood the symptoms may come and go and can affect different parts of the body at different times. In your case, the nerves that regulate the activity of your bowels have been affected. This is a distressing condition particularly as the diarrhoea often occurs at night. It may respond to a short course of antibiotics, which can be repeated if the diarrhoea returns. Standard diarrhoea treatments such as loperamide may be helpful. Irritable bowel syndrome can cause symptoms not unlike this – although it has nothing to do with diabetes. If you ever see blood or mucus in your stools, you should seek medical advice without delay.

> *I have had diabetes for more than 30 years and have had a lot of problems with vomiting recently. This has made my blood sugar levels rather unpredictable. Is there an explanation for this?*

In people who have had diabetes for many years, vomiting can be caused by a condition called gastroparesis. This results from damage to the nerves supplying the stomach (autonomic neuropathy). It is not uncommon for people to vomit food eaten several hours earlier because the stomach becomes paralysed and floppy and the food does not move through the digestive system in the normal way. This can lead to unpredictable blood sugar levels because the food is absorbed slowly and erratically. If you suffer from this condition it may be a good idea to delay your insulin injection until after you have eaten and your blood sugar has started to rise. It may be helped by anti-vomiting tablets such as metoclopramide.

> *The calf muscle in one leg seems to be shrinking. There is no ache and no pain. Is this anything to do with diabetes? I have been taking insulin for 15 years.*

You do not mention whether you have noticed any weakness in this leg. Occasionally diabetic neuropathy can affect the nerves which supply the muscles, causing the muscle to become weak and shrink in size without any accompanying pain or discomfort. It sounds as if this may be your problem.

I have had diabetes for many years and have developed
pain in my legs. My thighs in particular are very weak and
wasted. I have been told that I have 'diabetic amyotrophy'.
Will it get better?

D iabetic amyotrophy is a rare condition causing pain and weakness of one or both legs and is due to damage to nerves. It usually
occurs when diabetes control is very poor, but occasionally affects
people with only slight elevation of the blood glucose. Strict control
of diabetes leads to its improvement but it may take up to two years
or so for it to settle. The nerves affected are usually those supplying
the thigh muscles, as in your case, which become wasted and weak.

HEART AND BLOOD VESSEL DISEASE

I have read that poor circulation in the feet is a problem for
people with diabetes. Is there any way I can improve my
circulation to avoid developing this?

N arrowing ('hardening') of the arteries is a normal part of
growing older – and the arteries to the feet can be affected by
this process, leading to poor circulation in the feet and legs. The
causes of arterial disease are not very well understood, but we know
that smoking and poor diabetes control make it worse. So if you have
diabetes and smoke cigarettes, the risk of bad circulation increases
greatly. The best advice is to stop smoking, control your blood glucose,
and keep active – regular exercise will encourage the circulation to
improve. If you are unfortunate enough to develop circulation problems your GP can refer you to a vascular surgeon to see if the arteries
can be unblocked. This can sometimes be done by inserting a tube
with a small balloon into the artery (angioplasty) or alternatively by
an operation to bypass the blockage.

I'm in my seventies and am worried that I might develop heart problems. I am already being treated for high blood pressure. Is heart disease likely?

Heart disease is up to five times more common in people with diabetes and goes hand in hand with high blood pressure, excess body weight and raised cholesterol. This group of risk factors is an important cause of premature death in people with diabetes. We know that controlling blood pressure, cholesterol and blood glucose can help to reduce the chances of developing heart disease and there are now recommended targets for blood pressure, cholesterol and blood glucose, which your GP or practice nurse should be helping you to achieve.

Recently I have had some pain in my chest. My doctor says it could be angina and wants me to see a heart specialist for tests. What is angina and what will these tests involve?

Angina is a heart pain which occurs when the blood supply to the heart is insufficient because of narrowing of the coronary arteries. It is usually brought on by exercise, because that is when the heart needs most blood, but if the narrowing of the arteries is very severe, it may happen at rest. If one of the arteries becomes completely blocked, this leads to a heart attack. It is sometimes possible to improve the coronary circulation, either by inserting a small tube called a stent or by an operation to bypass the blockage.

The heart specialist may want to carry out various tests which may include asking you to walk on a treadmill while recording your heart tracing. He or she may also want to inject dye into the coronary arteries to identify the site of the blockage. This is normally done by inserting a tube into your groin area using a local anaesthetic. If it is not possible to correct the blockage, there are a number of treatments available which can widen the coronary arteries and prevent blood clots.

My husband died recently from a heart attack. He had had diabetes for 12 years and was controlled on tablets, and at about the same time that he developed diabetes he started having angina attacks. I wondered whether these were related and whether poor control had anything to do with his fatal heart attack?

There is certainly a connection between heart disease and diabetes. It has been shown that control of high blood pressure, cholesterol and blood glucose are all effective in preventing heart disease.

I am in my early twenties, but haven't had good diabetes control for a couple of years. Will this affect my arteries in later life?

It is unlikely to have much effect at your age but if you continue to have poor control over the next few years, you are likely to build up trouble for the future. Our arteries get more rigid and more clogged up as we get older and this process can be aggravated by periods of poor diabetes control and by smoking.

My left leg has been amputated because I developed diabetic gangrene. I now get a lot of pain in my right foot and calf. Could too much insulin be the cause of this pain?

It sounds as if the blood supply to your leg is insufficient and that this is the cause of the pain in your right foot and calf. As you know, this is the reason you developed gangrene in your left leg and you must be very worried about your right leg. You should tell your doctor about the pain as you may need to be referred to a vascular surgeon to see if anything can be done to improve the blood supply to your foot (see first question in this section).

There are a number of things you can do to help protect your remaining leg and these include:

- stopping smoking (if you smoke);

- keeping diabetes, blood pressure and cholesterol under very good control;

- maintaining close contact with a podiatrist who has a special interest in diabetes.

If you notice any sign of increased pain or change in colour, you should seek medical advice immediately.

My husband is 58 and has just been found to have diabetes when he went into hospital with a bad attack of angina. He has made a good recovery but has been sent home taking 4 insulin injections a day. I thought that in older people, insulin was only used when other treatments failed.

It was shown several years ago that if someone with diabetes had a heart attack and was treated intensively with insulin, they had a much better outcome with regard to their heart than those who were treated with tablets. The benefit was greatest in those people whose diabetes was discovered when they had the heart attack. This idea has been widely accepted and anyone with diabetes (previously known or not) who has a heart attack should receive an insulin infusion for 24 hours and when their heart problem is stable, they should go home on insulin for 3 months. This approach appears to provide long-lasting protection to the heart and, after three months, they can usually be changed to tablet treatment for their diabetes.

BLOOD PRESSURE

Now I have been diagnosed with diabetes, will I be more prone to high blood pressure and strokes?

Yes, there seems to be a very strong link between Type 2 diabetes and high blood pressure. Unfortunately both increase the risk of a stroke. The good news is that strict control of both diabetes and blood pressure keeps down this risk. Since publication of the UKPDS findings, we realise that if you have diabetes the blood pressure should be kept below 140/80. This may mean taking a combination of tablets and it is not unusual for people to require three or four different types of blood pressure tablets to achieve this target. The UKPDS research is described in the introduction to Chapter 4.

I have been told that my blood pressure is raised as a result of diabetic kidney problems and, because of this, it is very important that I take tablets to lower it – why is this?

There is good evidence to show that lowering the blood pressure to normal protects the kidneys from further damage. We also know that controlling blood pressure reduces the risk of heart disease and stroke. Studies in Germany and the UK have shown that blood pressure can be reduced significantly if people participate actively by self-monitoring of blood pressure. In these studies, participants were provided with a blood pressure monitor and given information about reducing high blood pressure; this included non-drug remedies, such as reducing salt, increasing fruit and vegetable intake and exercising. They were taught how to use an individual flow chart so they could make their own decisions about medication. The British Hypertension Society (address in Appendix 2) provides advice on how to select a reliable monitor, and if you think that you may benefit from self-monitoring of blood pressure, you should discuss this with your doctor or nurse.

I have been suffering from dizzy spells recently and on a couple of occasions I have fainted after standing up suddenly. My doctor says that this may be due to low blood pressure as a result of diabetes but I thought that diabetes caused high blood pressure. Can you explain?

Dizziness on standing up, sometimes known as postural hypotension, can be caused by autonomic neuropathy, when damage to the nerves controlling the blood pressure prevents the body from adjusting to changes in posture. This can lead to a rapid fall in blood pressure, most noticeable when you are standing up. The problem is made worse by poor control of diabetes, which can lead to dehydration. You should try to make sure that your diabetes is well controlled and if the problem persists you should see your GP. A tablet called fludrocortisone, which leads to fluid retention, can often help this condition.

THE MIND

I had a brain haemorrhage 18 months ago. Could this have been caused by my diabetes?

Brain haemorrhages and strokes are more common in people with diabetes, particularly if blood pressure levels are high. Since you have already had a stroke, you may be more at risk of other circulatory problems. This makes it particularly important that the usual risk factors (blood pressure, cholesterol and blood glucose) are kept under tight control. There is recent evidence that taking a high dose of a statin to reduce the cholesterol to very low levels has an additional benefit in lowering the risk of further stroke. Your doctor and diabetes nurse will be keen to help you with this.

I have been very depressed since my diagnosis. Are people
with diabetes more prone to depression?

Having to deal with the many demands of diabetes is bound to
cause you to feel gloomy at times and this seems to be most likely
when it hits home that you have diabetes for life with no chance of
a holiday from it. When large populations have been studied, the
frequency of depression in diabetes is about twice as common as in
people without the condition. Many people in your position find that
speaking to others in the same boat is helpful and this is one of the
positive features of the DESMOND programme (see p. 27). It is worth
making contact with the local branch of Diabetes UK.

I have read that hypos can cause brain damage – is this true?

It is possible for a severe hypo leading to unconsciousness for hours
or days to cause permanent brain damage. However, this cannot
result from 'normal' hypos that occur in the course of living with
diabetes and insulin. In practice, brain damage only occurs when
someone on insulin takes a deliberate overdose as a suicide attempt.
The tragic consequence of a failed attempt on one's life by insulin
overdose is that it can lead to severe brain damage and a life of
complete dependence on others.

There is also a suspicion that people who have repeated hypos for
20 or 30 years may have a form of memory loss late in life. However,
this is only conjecture and has never been proved.

9 | Research and the future

New developments and improvements in existing treatments can occur only through research; therefore research is vital to every person with diabetes. In the UK, Diabetes UK spends large sums (approximately £5 million each year) on research into diabetes. Members of local branches of Diabetes UK put a lot of energy into fundraising for the benefit of everyone with diabetes. There is always a need for more money because there are many good research ideas which are not funded. Other grant-giving bodies, such as the Medical Research Council and the Wellcome Trust contribute large sums to diabetes research. At the time of writing, it costs about £30,000 to support a relatively junior research worker for just one year.

The most inspiring research project in diabetes was the discovery of insulin itself in 1921, when a doctor and a medical student (Banting and Best) worked together during a few summer months to produce a life-saving treatment. There have been many important but less dramatic discoveries since then, each in some way contributing to our understanding of diabetes and many improving the available treatment.

Look at the Diabetes UK website for details of Diabetes UK research activities (see Appendix 2).

SEARCHING FOR CAUSES AND CURES

Do you think that diabetes will ever be cured?

Ever since a life-saving treatment for diabetes became available in 1922, there has been a constant search for a cure, which would relieve people of the burden of living with this condition. Great advances have been made in our understanding of the causes of Type 1 and Type 2 diabetes and at times it has looked as if a cure was just around the corner. Sadly these were false dawns but a huge amount of research effort continues to be devoted to trying to find a cure.

Will it ever be possible to prevent diabetes with a vaccine?

There is some evidence to suggest that certain virus infections can cause diabetes but we are not clear how often this happens: it is probably very infrequently. If a virus were isolated, which was found to cause diabetes, it would then be possible to produce a vaccine that could be given to children like the polio vaccine, to prevent them from developing diabetes later in life. At present this possibility seems rather remote.

TRANSPLANTATION

We have included this section to give information on a topic of great interest to people with diabetes. However, at the present time transplantation is not an effective treatment for Type 2 diabetes.

I should like to volunteer to have a pancreas transplant. Is there someone I must apply to? How successful have these operations been?

Pancreatic transplantation is not carried out in Type 2 diabetes and is still in the experimental stages for people with Type 1 diabetes. Technically, pancreatic transplants are even more difficult than liver, kidney or heart transplants. The pancreas is very delicate but also produces digestive juices, which digest the pancreas itself if it is damaged while being taken from the donor and placed in the recipient. The duct or tube through which these juices pass is narrow, and has to be joined up to the intestines in an intricate way so that the enzymes do not leak. Even if the procedure is a technical success, the body will still reject the transplant unless powerful drugs are given to suppress the immune system. Some of these (particularly steroids) tend to cause diabetes or make existing diabetes worse. Some UK transplant centres will offer people with diabetes who need a kidney transplant the chance to have a pancreas transplant at the same time. In these circumstances, the results seem to be better than if a pancreas is transplanted on its own. If both transplants are successful, this is a real bonus as the recipient can stop both renal dialysis and insulin. For those who do not have kidney failure, the most promising development is an islet cell transplant (see next question).

Are there any hospitals carrying out transplants of the islets of Langerhans? My daughter has Type 2 diabetes and I would like to help her.

Seven centres around the UK have signed up to the Diabetes UK Islet Transplantation Consortium but this group is only working on Type 1 diabetes. They hope to replicate and refine the technique developed by the English surgeon, James Shapiro, and his team in Edmonton, Canada. The Edmonton team took islet cells from donor pancreases and injected them into the liver of people with Type 1 diabetes. Once in the liver the cells developed a blood supply and began producing insulin. The entire transplantation process is now known as the Edmonton Protocol.

However, it is not possible to take islets from living donors so you would be unable to donate your cells to your daughter. This technique is still in the experimental stage but the results look promising. In Edmonton, 13 out of 15 islet cell transplants were 100% successful. With time, the transplanted islets began to fail so that after one year, 33% of patients needed insulin and by two years this figure was 57%. However, the transplants retain some capacity to produce insulin since most patients needed to take much lower doses of insulin after the procedure. The CITR website: spitfire.emmes.com/study/isl/index carries all this information.

Like transplantation of any other organ, an islet cell transplant requires powerful drugs to prevent rejection of the new cells (immunosuppressive therapy). As a result only people who have extreme problems in controlling their blood glucose levels are considered for transplantation. People who receive islet cell transplants need life-long immunosuppressive drugs, which may cause long-term side effects, including various forms of cancer.

Researchers have tried to prevent the need for immunosuppressant drugs by placing the islets in a small capsule which can resist rejection while allowing insulin to pass across the membrane. Unfortunately, after a time, the membrane tends to get clogged with scar tissue and the islet graft stops working.

Until there has been a major breakthrough in the transplantation of tissues from one individual to another, the hazards of long-term immunosuppressive therapy for someone receiving either a pancreas transplant or an islet cell transplant are greater than those of having diabetes treated with insulin. The problems are not insuperable but much more research needs to be done before transplantation becomes routine treatment for Type 1 diabetes.

NEW TREATMENTS

I have heard that some new drugs are becoming available for treatment of diabetes. Can you tell me something about these?

There is class of drugs known as PKC inhibitors which are in development and it is hoped they will protect against long-term complications. Protein kinase C is an enzyme which becomes activated by high blood glucose levels and causes damage to the lining of small blood vessels. We know that this type of damage is implicated in the development of some of the complications of diabetes, leading to changes in the retina, kidney and nerves. A class of drugs called PKC inhibitors blocks the action of protein kinase C and protects against diabetic complications. These treatments have been tested in people with retinopathy, nephropathy (kidney damage) and neuropathy (nerve damage) and the initial results are promising. Further testing is required before the drugs can be licensed for general use but it does look as though they will have a place in reversing the effect of some of the complications of diabetes.

I have Type 2 diabetes and have a constant battle with my weight. I am told that there is a new treatment which can help people to lose weight. Is this true?

There is a new class of drug called a GLP-1 agonist, which is taken by injection and can help people lose weight and control their diabetes. See page 61.

POSSIBLE DEVELOPMENTS IN INSULIN DELIVERY

What advances can we expect in the development of new insulin in the coming years?

Over the past 20 years, the range of insulins available has undergone a huge change and biosynthetic insulins have replaced the original animal insulins. There is more detail about human insulins in Chapter 3. They are manufactured by interfering with the genetic codes of bacteria and yeasts and inserting material that 'instructs' the organisms to produce insulin. By inserting the genetic material which codes for human insulin, scientists can persuade the organisms to produce human insulin. They can even get them to make 'new' analogue insulins with 'invented' structures – we are now in the era of 'designer' insulins! There is virtually unlimited capability to modify natural insulin and we expect to be able to develop a whole range of insulins with new properties that should improve therapy.

We are already beginning to see the benefits from this advance in scientific manufacturing. Analogue insulins with very rapid action are now widely used: Humalog® from Lilly and NovoRapid® from Novo Nordisk (see Table 3.1 in Chapter 3). Very long-acting analogues, Lantus® (Aventis) and Levemir® (Novo Nordisk) are now well-established.

Scientists are also looking for variations in the structure of the insulin which will 'target' the insulin more directly to the liver, the major organ responsible for glucose production in the body. Normally insulin is produced by the pancreas and goes directly to the liver but unfortunately, when people inject insulin, it has to pass through the lungs and other parts of the body before reaching the liver. It should be possible to modify the structure so that it can be targeted at the liver and control blood glucose more effectively.

I have heard that it is possible to get away from insulin injections either by using nasal insulin sprays or some form of insulin that can be taken by mouth. Are these claims true and are we going to be able to get away from insulin injections in the future?

There is no doubt that insulin delivered via the nose is absorbed through the mucous membranes and can lower the blood glucose. Unfortunately, only a small percentage of insulin taken in this manner is absorbed into the bloodstream and it is therefore an inefficient, unpredictable and expensive way of administering insulin.

If insulin is taken orally it is digested in the stomach and becomes inactive. It is possible to prevent this by incorporating insulin into a fat droplet (liposome), which enables it to be absorbed from the gut without being broken down by the digestive juices. However, the absorption is very erratic and there is no way of knowing when the insulin will be released from the droplet and become active.

Inhaled insulin (Exubera® made by Pfizer) became available in the UK in 2006 (see question under **Types of insulin** in Chapter 3). Unfortunately Exubera was withdrawn in 2008 because of lack of uptake and doubts about its safety. It seems unlikely that any other form of inhaled insulin will become available.

All these developments are exciting but there are various issues to be aware of when considering the effectiveness of inhaled and oral insulin.

- People must be confident of receiving an accurate dose of the insulin.

- Inhalers often use very large doses of insulin.

- We do not yet know the potential side effects of such large doses.

- The inhalers being developed so far do not totally eliminate the need for insulin injections.

- The devices need to be portable, compact and competitively priced.

INSULIN PUMPS AND ARTIFICIAL PANCREAS

I recently read about a device called a 'glucose sensor', which can control the insulin administered to animals with diabetes. Will this ever be used on humans and if so what can we expect from it?

Research has been going on for many years into the development of a small electronic device that could be implanted under the skin and continuously monitor the level of glucose in the blood. The technical problems of such a device are considerable and it seems unlikely to be used routinely in people with diabetes for several years. Not only are there technical problems in achieving an accurate reflection of blood glucose level by an implanted glucose sensor, but there is also the major problem of 'hooking it up' to a supply of insulin to be released according to the blood glucose level. Clinical trials are being carried out in the USA and France using an intravenous glucose sensor in conjunction with an implantable pump. The early results are encouraging, but it will be several years before it is widely available.

I understand that there are ways of testing blood glucose without pricking the skin. Can you tell me more about them?

There are regular reports in the press about 'non-invasive' blood glucose monitoring devices being developed. Some of these devices are not totally non-invasive. One involves a needle being inserted under the skin for up to three days at a time so that blood glucose readings can be taken every few minutes. At the moment the readings given can be accessed only by a healthcare professional, but it is hoped that eventually people will be able to read these results for themselves. This method of monitoring could be useful if the device were attached to an insulin pump adjusting the amount of insulin administered in response to the blood glucose level. Although this is not yet possible, it is likely to be developed in the near future.

I hear that there are pumps available that can be implanted like pacemakers – is this true? What are the likely developments with insulin pumps within the next five years?

Yes, it is true that insulin pumps have been implanted into people as part of research studies and there has been some encouraging progress in this field. Although still experimental and a long way from being a standard form of treatment, there are pumps small enough to be implanted into the wall of the abdomen, where they remain for several years. One such pump is made by MiniMed but is very expensive and not available in the UK or USA. The pump does not have a sensor to detect glucose but simply provides background insulin at a rate that can be regulated from the outside using a small radio transmitter. This device can be used to infuse more insulin before a meal. There is a reservoir of insulin that has to be refilled through the skin with a syringe and needle but changing the batteries requires a small operation. Although it looks promising, this device is complex and expensive and remains a research procedure.

I have heard about the artificial pancreas or 'Biostator'.
Apparently this machine is capable of maintaining blood
glucose at normal levels, irrespective of what is eaten.
Is this true? If so, why isn't it widely available?

The Biostator is an artificial pancreas, which measures the blood glucose concentration continuously and infuses insulin at a rate which keeps the blood glucose normal. Unfortunately these machines are the size of a domestic washing machine and are technically complex. Their major value is for research purposes since they are quite unsuitable at present as devices for long-term control. The Biostator has been around for 30 years and throughout this time, bioengineering groups have tried but failed to reduce it to a size that would be practical for everyday use.

10 | Self-help groups

This chapter describes the various organisations that have grown up to help people with diabetes.

People react in different ways to being diagnosed with diabetes: some will become withdrawn, while others will set out to gather as much information as possible. Whatever your reaction, you should make contact with Diabetes UK, where you will come across people who are living with diabetes and who have learned to cope with many of the daily problems. These people and the staff at Diabetes UK should provide an extra dimension to the information that you have been given by doctors, nurses, dietitians and other professionals.

DIABETES UK

This organisation was founded in 1934, under the name of the British Diabetic Association, by two people with diabetes, the author H G Wells and R D Lawrence, a doctor based at the diabetes clinic of King's College Hospital, London. In a letter to *The Times* dated January 1933, they announced their intention to set up an 'association open to all diabetics, rich or poor, for mutual aid and assistance, and to promote the study, the diffusion of knowledge, and the proper treatment of diabetes in this country'. They proposed that people with diabetes, members of the general public interested in diabetes, and doctors and nurses should be persuaded to join the projected association. Over 70 years later Diabetes UK is a credit to its founders.

In many countries there are separate organisations for people with diabetes and for professionals, but Diabetes UK draws its strength from the fact that both interest groups are united in the same society. Diabetes UK is the largest organisation in the UK working for people with diabetes, funding research, campaigning, and helping people live with the condition. The Careline offers confidential support and information on all aspects of diabetes (0845 120 2960, Monday–Friday, 9 a.m.–5 p.m.). During 2006 Careline handled an average of 200 calls each day. In order to make Careline accessible to all, there is access to an interpreting service.

Many people with diabetes experience discrimination when taking out insurance by way of increased premiums, restricted terms or even downright refusal. Faced with the general lack of understanding within the insurance market, Diabetes UK has negotiated its own exclusive schemes to provide policies suited to the needs of people with diabetes and those living with them. Diabetes UK Insurance Services offers competitively priced home and motor, travel and personal finance products. For more details telephone 0800 731 7431 (or email diabetes@heathlambert.com).

Up-to-date information and news is published in Balance, a magazine that appears every other month. *Diabetes for beginners* is provided for newly diagnosed people, both Type 1 and Type 2 (insulin dependent and non-insulin dependent). Diabetes UK produces its own leaflets and books, and also sells books produced by other publishers (see Appendix 1). Diabetes UK has an excellent website (www.diabetes. org.uk) where you can find out more information about the work of charity and how they can help you. Diabetes UK's address is given in Appendix 2.

Joining Diabetes UK

Diabetes UK works to influence the decisions made about living with diabetes, and the more members it has, the greater its influence. Diabetes UK cannot continue to provide its services and activities to all people with diabetes without your support. If you would like more information about joining Diabetes UK, call 0845 123 2399 or write to Diabetes UK at the address shown in Appendix 2.

Diabetes UK Local Support Groups

There are nearly 400 voluntary groups and parents' groups throughout the country. These are run entirely by volunteers and, because of their commitment, large sums of money are raised for research into diabetes. Diabetes UK branches also aim to increase public awareness of diabetes, and arrange meetings for local people with diabetes and their families for support and information.

Diabetes UK holidays

The first diabetes holidays for children in the UK took place in 1935 and running these holidays has grown into a large enterprise. During the summer of 2006, at seven different sites throughout the UK, 250 children aged 7–18 years enjoyed a week away with Diabetes UK. These educational holidays are organised by the Care Support team, and they give the opportunity for children to meet others with diabetes and to become more independent of their parents. They aim to give the children a good time, encourage them to try new activities, while at the same time teaching them more about their diabetes and giving their parents a well-earned break.

Diabetes UK family weekends

The Care Support team also organises family weekends for parents of children with diabetes. These cater for about 200 families each year. While parents have talks and discussions from specialist doctors, nurses and dietitians, there are activities for children throughout the weekend supervised by skilled and experienced helpers.

Diabetes UK adult support weekends

These weekends are for adults with diabetes who have been diagnosed in the last two or three years. They offer a chance for people with Type 1 or Type 2 diabetes to meet others, join in discussion groups, talk to healthcare professionals, and learn more about healthy eating, exercise and care.

JUVENILE DIABETES RESEARCH FOUNDATION (JDRF)

This organisation was founded in 1970 by a small group of parents of children with diabetes. The Juvenile Diabetes Research Foundation exists to find a cure for diabetes and its complications. They support diabetes worldwide and provide research funds at a comparable level to Diabetes UK. The address and website can be found in Appendix 2.

INSULIN-PUMPERS UK

This group was formed to raise funds and provide information on insulin pumps. The website address can be found in Appendix 2.

INSULIN DEPENDENT DIABETES TRUST (IDDT)

This is a registered charity formed in 1994, which is concerned with listening to the needs of people who live with diabetes. The aims of the Trust are:

- to offer care and support to people with diabetes and their carers, especially those experiencing difficulties with genetically engineered 'human' insulin;

- to influence appropriate bodies to ensure that a wide range of insulins remains available, to ensure that all insulin users have a continued supply of their chosen insulin;

- to ensure that all people with diabetes and carers are properly informed of the various treatments available to them, as is their right under the Patients' Charter;

- to collect information and experiences from people with diabetes and their carers to help others in the same situation and to pass it to healthcare professionals to create a better understanding of 'life with diabetes';

- where possible, to represent the direct voice of the person with diabetes, as the consumer, in relation to healthcare and research.

The Trust is run entirely by voluntary donations and does not accept funding from the pharmaceutical industry, in order to remain uninfluenced and independent. The address and website can be found in Appendix 2.

NATIONAL KIDNEY FEDERATION (NKF)

The NKF is a UK-wide charity run by kidney patients for kidney patients. While it used to be concerned almost solely with people with advanced or end-stage renal failure, there is much more emphasis now also on people at earlier stages of kidney disease. If you have even a mild form of kidney disease, the NKF can help you find information and support to keep your kidneys as healthy as possible for as long as possible.

One of the long-term complications of diabetes can be some degree of kidney damage, so it is important for people with diabetes to be aware of this organisation and what it has to offer. The address and website can be found in Appendix 2.

11 | Emergencies

This chapter is for quick reference if things are going badly wrong. It includes vital information for people who have diabetes, as well as some simple rules for relatives and friends. These rules are designed to be consulted in an emergency, although it would be worth looking through them before you are faced with a crisis. You can read more about hypos on p. 101 and about how to deal with illness on p. 164. It seems a pity to end this book in such a negative way by telling you what to do in an emergency. We hope that by keeping your diabetes well controlled you will avoid these serious situations.

The advice is mainly for people taking insulin. If your diabetes is treated with tablets and your blood sugar level is high, consult your doctor. It may be possible to increase your tablets, but in some circumstances you may need insulin to tide you over the illness. This sometimes means admission to hospital.

People taking tablets are not as likely to become hypo (low blood sugar) as those taking insulin, but it can happen (see the section

Hypos in Chapter 3). The warning signs and treatment are the same as for people taking insulin, but as it may take longer for the effect of tablets to wear off, it is important to check the blood glucose every 2–3 hours, until you are certain the hypo will not return. If you are having regular hypos, speak to your doctor or practice nurse as your tablets may need to be reduced.

Elderly people are prone to confusion if their blood glucose is low and may need admission to hospital for close observation until their sugar is normal.

WHAT EVERY PERSON ON INSULIN MUST KNOW

- Never stop insulin if you feel ill or sick. Illness often causes a rise in blood sugar and you may need more rather than less insulin even if you are not eating. Check your blood sugar frequently and take extra short-acting insulin every 3–4 hours if you are high. Be prepared with a high sugar drink such as Lucozade so that if you do go low you can correct it quickly.

- If you do not have any short-acting insulin, contact your doctor.

- If you are being sick, try to keep up a good fluid intake – at least 2½ litres (4 pints) a day. If you are unable to keep down fluids, you will need to go to hospital for an intravenous drip.

- Always keep sugar or some similar quick-acting carbohydrate on your person.

- Never risk driving if your blood sugar could be low. People with diabetes do lose their driving licence if found at the wheel when hypo.

- Remember physical exercise and alcohol are both likely to bring on a hypo.

WHAT OTHER PEOPLE MUST KNOW ABOUT DIABETES

- Never stop insulin in case of sickness (no apologies for repeating this). Check blood sugar regularly and keep a glucose drink nearby in case of hypo. Be prepared to use extra insulin if the blood tests are high.

- Repeated vomiting, drowsiness and laboured breathing are serious warning signs in someone with diabetes. They suggest impending coma and can only be treated in hospital.

- A person who is hypo may not be in full command of their senses and may take a lot of persuasion to have some sugar. Jam or a sugary drink (e.g. Lucozade) may be easier to get down than Dextro-Energy tablets. Glucogel (previously known as Hypostop) which can be absorbed through the cheeks or gums may be useful.

- Never let someone drive if you suspect they are hypo. It could be fatal.

FOODS TO EAT IN AN EMERGENCY OR WHEN FEELING UNWELL

Each of the following contains 10 g carbohydrate.

- 100 mL pure fruit juice
- 100 mL cola (not *diet* cola)
- 60 mL Lucozade
- small scoop ice-cream
- two sugar cubes or two teaspoons of sugar
- one ordinary jelly cube or two heaped tablespoons of made-up jelly
- 200 mL (about ½ pint) of milk
- small bowl of thickened soup
- two cream crackers
- one natural yoghurt
- one diet fruit yoghurt
- one apple or pear or orange
- one small banana
- three Dextro-Energy tablets

If you are feeling unwell, eating solid foods may not be possible and you may need to rely on sweet fluids to provide the necessary carbohydrate. Liquids such as cold, defizzed (allowed to stand and go flat) Coca-Cola or Lucozade are useful if you feel sick. Do not worry about eating the exact amount of carbohydrate at the correct time but as a general rule try to eat little and often.

If you continue to vomit, *seek medical advice*.

SIGNS AND SYMPTOMS OF HYPOGLYCAEMIA

This is *low* blood sugar, also called a hypo, a reaction or an insulin reaction. The following signs and symptoms can develop over minutes.

- Trembling
- Sweating
- Tingling of the lips and tongue
- Weakness
- Tiredness
- Sleepiness
- Hunger
- Blurred vision
- Palpitations
- Nausea
- Headache
- Mental confusion
- Unsteadiness
- Pallor
- Slurred speech
- Bad temper
- Change in behaviour
- Lack of concentration
- Unconsciousness (hypoglycaemic or insulin coma)

If possible treat the low sugar with a sweet drink followed by some food such as biscuits or a sandwich. If the person is unable to swallow, a glucagon injection may be needed. If in doubt, dial 999 and ask for paramedic help. Tablets may sometimes lead to recurrent or prolonged hypos. Hospital admission may be required.

SIGNS AND SYMPTOMS OF HYPERGLYCAEMIA

This is *high* blood sugar. The following signs and symptoms develop over hours.

- Thirst
- Excess urine
- Nausea
- Abdominal pain
- Vomiting
- Drowsiness
- Rapid breathing
- Flushed, dry skin
- Unconsciousness (hyperglycaemic or diabetic coma)

A high blood sugar in someone who feels perfectly well is not a cause for concern. If necessary, extra short-acting insulin can be taken to bring the blood sugar down. If your blood sugar remains high after taking extra insulin, and you are feeling unwell, you may need to be treated in hospital with fluids and insulin given into a vein. If you are worried, seek medical advice. Drowsiness, rapid breathing or unconsciousness are very serious signs and medical help should be obtained immediately.

Glossary

Terms in *italics* in these definitions refer to other terms in the glossary.

acarbose A drug that slows the digestion and absorption of complex *carbohydrates*.

Acesulfane-K A low-*calorie* intense sweetener.

acetone One of the chemicals called *ketones* formed when the body uses up fat for energy. The presence of acetone in the urine usually means that more insulin is needed.

adrenaline A hormone produced by the adrenal glands, which prepares the body for action (the 'flight or fight' reaction) and also increases the level of blood glucose. Produced by the body in response to many stimuli including a low blood glucose.

albumin A protein present in most animal tissues. The presence of albumin in the urine may denote kidney damage or be simply due to a urinary infection.

alpha cell The cell that produces *glucagon* – found in the *islets of Langerhans* in the pancreas.

alpha glucosidase inhibitor A tablet that slows the digestion of carbohydrates in the intestine (acarbose).

analogue insulin Insulin that has the molecular structure changed to alter its action.

angiography A special type of X-ray where dye is injected into an artery to detect narrowing.

angioplasty A technique which uses an inflatable balloon to widen narrowed arteries.

antigens Proteins which the body recognises as 'foreign' and which trigger an immune response.

arteriosclerosis or **arterial sclerosis** or **arterial disease** Hardening of the arteries: loss of elasticity in the walls of the arteries from thickening and calcification. Occurs with advancing years in those with or without diabetes. May affect the heart (causing thrombosis), the brain (a stroke) or the circulation to the legs and feet.

aspartame A low-calorie intense sweetener. Brand name NutraSweet®.

autonomic neuropathy Damage to the system of nerves regulating many automatic functions of the body such as stomach emptying, sexual function (potency) and blood pressure control.

bacteria A type of germ.

balanitis Inflammation of the end of the penis, usually caused by yeast infections as a result of sugar in the urine.

beta-blockers Drugs that block the effect of stress hormones on the cardiovascular system. Often used to treat angina and to lower blood pressure. May change the warning signs of *hypoglycaemia*.

beta cell The cell that produces insulin – found in the *islets of Langerhans* in the *pancreas*.

biguanides A group of antidiabetes tablets that lower blood glucose levels. Their mode of action is not well understood but they work in part by increasing the body's sensitivity to insulin. Metformin is the only preparation in this group.

blood glucose monitoring System of measuring blood glucose levels at home using a portable meter and reagent sticks.

bran Indigestible husk of the wheat grain. A type of *dietary fibre*.

brittle diabetes Refers to diabetes that is very unstable with swings from very low to very high blood glucose levels and often involving frequent admissions to hospital.

calories Units in which energy or heat are measured. The energy value of food is measured in calories.

carbohydrates A class of food that comprises starches and sugars and is most readily available by the body for energy. Found mainly in plant foods. Examples are rice, bread, potatoes, pasta and beans.

cataract Opacity of the lens of the eye, which obscures vision. It may be removed surgically.

CEMACH Confidential Enquiry into Maternal and Child Health. An audit of pregnancy outcome in mothers with diabetes.

Charcot foot Swelling of the foot, sometimes leading to deformity, as a result of lack of sensation (neuropathy).

clear insulin The term used to refer to short-acting insulins. However, the two long-acting analogue insulins (Lantus® and Levemir®) are also clear so the term must be used with caution.

cloudy insulin Longer-acting insulin with fine particles of insulin bound to protamine or zinc.

coma A form of unconsciousness from which people can be roused only with difficulty. If caused by diabetes, may be a *diabetic coma* or an *insulin coma*.

complications Long-term consequences of imperfectly controlled diabetes. For details see Chapter 8.

control Usually refers to blood glucose control. The aim of good control is to achieve normal blood glucose levels (4–10 mmol/L) and HbA$_{1c}$ less than 7%.

coronary heart disease Disease of the blood vessels supplying the heart.

cystitis Inflammation of the bladder, which usually causes frequent passing of urine, accompanied by a burning pain.

DAFNE Dose Adjustment For Normal Eating. An intensive education programme for people with Type 1 diabetes.

DESMOND Diabetes Education and Self Management Ongoing and Newly Diagnosed. An education programme for people with Type 2 diabetes.

detemir A new insulin analogue designed to last for 24 hours and act as basal insulin. Also called Levemir®.

Dextro-Energy Glucose tablets.

diabetes insipidus A disorder of the pituitary gland accompanied by excessive urination and thirst. Nothing to do with *diabetes mellitus*.

diabetes mellitus A disorder of the pancreas characterised by a high blood glucose level. This book is about diabetes mellitus.

diabetic amyotrophy Rare condition causing pain and/or weakness of the legs from the damage to certain nerves.

diabetic coma Extreme form of *hyperglycaemia*, usually with *ketoacidosis*, causing unconsciousness.

diabetic diarrhoea A form of diabetic *autonomic neuropathy* leading to diarrhoea.

diabetic foods Food products targeted at people with diabetes, in which ordinary sugar (sucrose) is replaced with substitutes such as *fructose* or *sorbitol*. These foods are not recommended as part of your food plan.

diabetic nephropathy Kidney damage that may occur in diabetes.

diabetic neuropathy Nerve damage that may occur in diabetes.

diabetic retinopathy Eye disease that may occur in diabetes.

dietary fibre Part of plant material that resists digestion and gives bulk to the diet. Also called fibre or roughage.

diuretics Agents that increase the flow of urine, commonly known as water tablets.

DPP4 inhibitors New generation of agents to treat Type 2 diabetes. DPP4 inhibitors (*gliptins*) can be taken in tablet form and work by slowing the breakdown of GLP-1.

epidural A type of anaesthetic commonly used in obstetrics. Anaesthetic solution is injected through the spinal canal to numb the lower part of the body.

erectile dysfunction Inability to achieve or maintain an erection (*impotence*).

fibre Another name for dietary fibre.

fructosamine Measurement of diabetes control that reflects the average blood glucose level over the previous 2–3 weeks. Similar to haemoglobin A_{1c} which averages the blood glucose over the longer period of 2–3 months.

fructose Type of sugar found naturally in fruit and honey. Since it does not require insulin for its metabolism, it is often used as a sweetener in diabetic foods.

gangrene Death of a part of the body due to a very poor blood supply. A combination of *neuropathy* and *arteriosclerosis* may lead to unrecognised injuries to the feet . If the injury becomes infected this can lead to gangrene in some circumstances.

gastroparesis Delayed emptying of the stomach as a result of autonomic neuropathy. Can lead to erratic food absorption and vomiting.

gestational diabetes Diabetes which is diagnosed during pregnancy.

glargine A new insulin analogue designed to last for 24 hours to act as basal (background) insulin. Also called Lantus®.

glaucoma Disease of the eye causing increased pressure inside the eyeball.

gliptins see *DPP4 inhibitors*.

glitazones A group of drugs that reduce *insulin resistance* – see *thiazolidinedione*.

GLP-1 Glucagon-like peptide – a hormone which increases the production of insulin in response to food. Two GLP-1 agents (exenatide or liraglutide) are available in the UK.

glucagon A hormone produced by the *alpha cells* in the pancreas which causes a rise in blood glucose by freeing *glycogen* from the liver. Available in injection form for use in treating a severe hypo.

glucose Form of sugar made by digestion of carbohydrates. Absorbed into the bloodstream where it circulates and is used as a source of energy.

glucose tolerance test Test used in the diagnosis of diabetes mellitus. The glucose in the blood is measured at intervals before and after the person has drunk a large amount of glucose whilst fasting.

glycogen The form in which carbohydrate is stored in the liver and muscles. It is often known as animal starch.

glycaemic index (GI) A way of describing how a carbohydrate-containing food affects blood glucose levels.

glycosuria Presence of glucose in the urine.

glycosylated haemoglobin Another name for haemoglobin A_{1c}.

haemoglobin A1c The part of the haemoglobin or colouring matter of the red blood cell which has glucose attached to it. A test of diabetes control. The amount of haemoglobin A_{1c} in the blood depends on the average blood glucose level over the previous 2–3 months.

honeymoon period Time when the dose of insulin drops shortly after starting insulin treatment. It is the result of partial recovery of insulin secretion by the pancreas. Usually the honeymoon period only lasts for a few months.

hormone Substance generated in one gland or organ which is carried by the blood to another part of the body to control another organ. Insulin and glucagon are both hormones.

human insulin Insulin that has been manufactured to be identical to that produced in the human pancreas. Differs slightly from older insulins, which were extracted from cows or pigs.

hydramnios An excessive amount of amniotic fluid, which is the fluid surrounding the baby before birth.

hyperglycaemia High blood glucose (above 10 mmol/L).

hypo Abbreviation for hypoglycaemia.

hypoglycaemia (also known as a hypo or an insulin reaction) Low blood glucose (below 3.5 mmol/L).

impotence Failure of erection of the penis. Also called *erectile dysfunction*.

injector Device to aid injections.

Innolet A simple injector for insulin designed for people with poor vision or problems with their hands such as arthritis.

insulin A hormone produced by the *beta cells* of the pancreas and responsible for control of blood glucose. Insulin can only be given by injection because digestive juices destroy its action if taken by mouth.

insulin coma Extreme form of *hypoglycaemia* associated with unconsciousness and sometimes convulsions.

insulin dependent diabetes (abbreviation IDD) Former name for Type 1 diabetes.

insulin pen Device that resembles a large fountain pen that takes a cartridge of insulin. The injection of insulin is given after dialling the dose and pressing a button that releases the insulin.

insulin reaction Another name for *hypoglycaemia* or a hypo. In America it is called an insulin shock.

insulin resistance A condition where the normal amount of insulin is not able to keep the blood glucose level down to normal. Such people need large doses of insulin to control their diabetes. The glitazone group of tablets is designed to reduce insulin resistance.

intermediate-acting insulin Insulin preparations with action lasting 12–18 hours.

intradermal Meaning 'into the skin'. Usually refers to an injection given into the most superficial layer of the skin. Insulin must not be given in this way as it is painful and will not be absorbed properly (see Figure 3.3).

intramuscular A deep injection into the muscle.

islets of Langerhans Specialised cells within the pancreas that produce *insulin* and *glucagon*.

isophane A form of intermediate-acting insulin that has protamine added to slow its absorption.

joule Unit of work or energy used in the metric system. A *calorie* is equivalent to about 4.18 joules. Some dietitians calculate food energy in joules.

juvenile-onset diabetes Outdated name for Type 1 diabetes, so-called because most patients who need insulin straight away develop diabetes under the age of 40. The term is no longer used because Type 1 diabetes can occur at any age, although more commonly in young people.

ketoacidosis A serious condition caused by lack of insulin which results in body fat being used up to form *ketones* and acids. Characterised by high blood glucose levels, ketones in the urine, vomiting, drowsiness, heavy laboured breathing and a smell of acetone on the breath.

ketones Acid substances (including acetone) formed when body fat is used up to provide energy.

ketonuria The presence of *acetone* and other ketones in the urine. Detected by testing with a special testing stick (Ketostix®, Ketur Test®). Presence of ketones in the urine is due to lack of insulin or periods of starvation.

laser treatment Process in which laser beams are used to treat a damaged retina (back of the eye). Used in *photocoagulation*.

lente insulin A form of intermediate-acting insulin that has zinc added to slow its absorption. It is now obsolete and very few people use this insulin.

lipoatrophy Loss of fat from injection sites. It used to occur before the use of highly purified insulins.

lipohypertrophy Fatty swelling usually caused by repeated injections of insulin into the same site.

maturity-onset diabetes Another term for Type 2 diabetes most commonly occurring in people who are middle-aged and overweight.

metabolic rate Rate of oxygen consumption by the body, rate at which you 'burn up' the food you eat.

metabolic syndrome A condition of people who have *insulin resistance* and are at extra risk of heart disease. Features include Type 2 diabetes, high cholesterol, raised blood pressure and central obesity. It may also be associated with polycystic ovary syndrome and fatty liver disease.

metabolism Process by which the body turns food into energy.

metformin A biguanide tablet that works by reducing the release of glucose from the liver and increasing the uptake of glucose into the muscle.

microalbuminuria Small amounts of protein in the urine, not detectable by dipstick for albumin (*proteinuria*). Raised levels indicate early kidney damage.

microaneurysms Small red dots on the retina at the back of the eye which are one of the earliest signs of diabetic *retinopathy*. Represent areas of weakness of the very small blood vessels in the eye. Microaneurysms do not affect the eyesight in any way.

micromole One-thousandth (1/1000) of a millimole.

millimole Unit for measuring the concentration of glucose and other substances in the blood. Blood glucose is measured in millimoles per litre (mmol/L). It has replaced milligrammes per decilitre (mg/dL or mg%) as a unit of measurement although this is still used in some other countries. 1 mmol/L = 18 mg/dL.

nateglinide A prandial glucose regulator.

nephropathy Kidney damage. In the first instance this makes the kidney more leaky so that *albumin* appears in the urine. At a later stage it may affect the function of the kidney and in severe cases lead to kidney failure.

neuropathy Damage to the nerves, which may be *peripheral* neuropathy or *autonomic neuropathy*. It can occur with diabetes especially when poorly controlled, but also has other causes.

NICE National Institute for Health and Clinical Excellence. An independent organisation providing national guidance to promote good health. It provides guidelines for the use of new and existing drugs in the NHS.

non-insulin dependent diabetes (abbreviation NIDD) Former name for Type 2 diabetes.

orlistat A tablet that blocks the digestion of fat. Brand name Xenical®. Used to help people lose weight, which in turn may improve control of diabetes.

pancreas Gland lying behind the stomach, which as well as secreting a digestive fluid (pancreatic juice) also produces the hormones *insulin* and *glucagon*. Contains *islets of Langerhans*.

peripheral neuropathy Damage to the nerves supplying the muscles and skin. This can result in diminished sensation, particularly in the feet and legs, and in muscle weakness. May also cause pain in the feet or legs.

phimosis Inflammation and narrowing of the foreskin of the penis.

photocoagulation Process of treating diabetic retinopathy with light beams, either laser beams or xenon arc. This technique focuses a beam of light on a very tiny area of the retina. This beam is so intense that it causes a very small burn, which may close off a leaking blood vessel or destroy weak blood vessels that are at risk of bleeding.

pioglitazone A tablet that targets insulin resistance. Trade name Actos®.

PKC inhibitors (protein kinase C inhibitors) Developed to try and reverse the changes in small blood vessels which cause diabetic eye disease (retinopathy). Though they seem to help in isolated cases, overall the results have been disappointing.

polydipsia Being excessively thirsty and drinking too much. It is a symptom of untreated diabetes.

polyuria The passing of large quantities of urine due to excess glucose from the bloodstream. It is a symptom of untreated diabetes.

pork insulin Insulin extracted from the pancreas of pigs.

prandial glucose regulators Tablets taken before meals that stimulate the release of insulin from the pancreas (repaglinide and nateglinide). Only used in Type 2 diabetes.

pre-eclampsia A condition which occurs towards the end of pregnancy and leads to high blood pressure, protein in the urine and in severe cases, convulsions. Pre-eclampsia normally resolves soon after delivery.

protein One of the classes of food that is necessary for growth and repair of tissues. Found in fish, meat, eggs, milk and pulses. Can also refer to albumin when found in the urine.

proteinuria Protein or albumin in the urine.

pruritus vulvae Irritation of the vulva (the genital area in women). Caused by an infection that occurs because of an excess of sugar in the urine and is often an early sign of diabetes in the older person. It clears up when the blood glucose levels return to normal and the sugar disappears from the urine.

pyelonephritis Inflammation and infection of the kidney.

renal threshold The level of glucose in the blood above which it will begin to spill into the urine. The usual renal threshold for glucose in the blood is about 10 mmol/L, so when the blood glucose rises above 10 mmol/L, glucose appears in the urine.

repaglinide A prandial glucose regulator.

retina Light-sensitive area at the back of the eye.

retinal screening Photograph of the retina to identify changes due to diabetes at a stage that they can be treated to prevent loss of vision. Usually carried out once a year.

retinopathy Damage to the retina.

rosiglitazone A tablet that targets insulin resistance. Trade names Avandia® and Avandamet® (in combination with metformin).

roughage Another name for dietary fibre.

saccharin A synthetic sweetener that is calorie free.

short-acting insulin Insulin preparations with action lasting 6–8 hours.

Snellen chart Chart showing rows of letters in decreasing sizes. Used for measuring visual acuity.

sorbitol A chemical related to sugar and alcohol that is used as a sweetening agent in foods as a substitute for ordinary sugar. It has no significant effect upon the blood glucose level but has the same number of calories as ordinary sugar so should not be used by those who need to lose weight. Poorly absorbed and may have a laxative effect.

steroids Hormones produced by the adrenal glands, testes and ovaries. Also available in synthetic form. Tend to increase the blood glucose level and make diabetes worse.

subcutaneous injection An injection beneath the skin into the layer of fat that lies between the skin and muscle. The normal way of giving insulin.

sucrose A sugar (containing glucose and fructose in combination) derived from sugar cane or sugar beet (i.e. ordinary table sugar). It is a pure carbohydrate.

sulphonylureas Antidiabetes tablets that lower the blood glucose by stimulating the pancreas to produce more insulin. Commonly used sulphonylureas are gliclazide and glibenclamide.

thiazolidenedione Generic name for group of tablets that target insulin resistance and improve diabetes in Type 2 diabetes. Pharmaceutical names are rosiglitazone and pioglitazone, brand names are Avandia® and Actos®.

thrombosis Clot forming in a blood vessel.

tissue markers Proteins on the outside of cells in the body that are genetically determined.

toxaemia Poisoning of the blood by the absorption of toxins. Usually refers to the toxaemia of pregnancy, which is characterised by high blood pressure, proteinuria and ankle swelling.

Type 1 diabetes Name for insulin dependent diabetes which cannot be treated by diet and tablets alone. Outdated name is juvenile-onset diabetes. Age of onset is usually below the age of 40 years.

Type 2 diabetes Name for non-insulin dependent diabetes. Age of onset is usually above the age of 40 years, often in people who are overweight. These people do not always need insulin treatment and can usually be successfully treated with diet alone or diet and tablets. Formerly known as maturity-onset diabetes.

U40 insulin The old weaker strength (40 units per ml) of insulin, no longer available in the UK. It is still available in Eastern Europe and in some countries in the Far East, such as Vietnam and Indonesia.

U100 insulin The standard strength (100 units per ml) of insulin in the UK, USA, Canada, Australia, New Zealand, South Africa, the Middle East and the Far East.

urine testing The detection of abnormal amounts of glucose, ketones, protein or blood in the urine, usually by means of urine testing sticks.

virus A very small organism capable of causing disease.

viscous fibre A type of dietary fibre found in pulses (peas, beans and lentils) and some fruit and vegetables.

visual acuity Acuteness of vision. Measured by reading letters on a sight testing chart (a Snellen chart).

water tablets The common name for diuretics.

Xenical® The brand name for orlistat.

Appendix 1: Publications

At the time of writing, all the publications listed here were available. Check with your local bookshop or Diabetes UK for current prices.

ABOUT DIABETES

Books

Type 2 Diabetes in Adults of All Ages, by Charles Fox and Ragnar Hanas. Class Publishing (2008)

Diabetes: A Practical Guide to Managing Your Health by Jill Rodgers and Rosemary Walker. Dorling Kindersley (2010)

Type 2 Diabetes: Your Questions Answered by Jill Rodgers and Rosemary Walker. Dorling Kindersley (2006)

Need to Know: Diabetes (Need to Know) by Jenny Bryan. Heinemann (2004)

Diabetes and Your Teenager by Bonnie Estridge and Jo Davies. Harper Collins (1996)

Magazines and booklets

These titles are all published by Diabetes UK.

Balance – Diabetes UK's own magazine which appears every other month

Diabetes for Beginners: Type 1

Diabetes for Beginners: Type 2

What Diabetes Care to Expect

Living Healthily with Diabetes- a guide for Black African-Caribbean communities

Coping with diabetes when you are ill

NUTRITION

Apart from the books listed here, you will also be able to find other titles in your local library or on Amazon.

Books

The Everyday Diabetic Cookbook by Stella Bowling. Grub Street Publishing (1995)

The Good Housekeeping Diabetic Cookbook by Azmina Govindji. Collins & Brown (2005)

Leaflets

These are available from Diabetes UK, some as downloads.

Food choices and diabetes

Eating well with diabetes

Alcohol and diabetes

Recipe books

These titles are all published by Diabetes UK.

The Diabetes Weight Loss Diet

Home Baking

Managing your weight – a balanced approach

Christmas and other celebrations

Quick cooking for diabetes

Appendix 2: Useful addresses

Abbotts Diabetes Care
Formerly MediSense Britain
Helpline: 0500 467466
www.abbottukdiabetescare.co.uk
*Manufactures blood glucose
monitoring systems and meters, and
provides information*

AccuChek
Customer careline: 0800 701 000
*Insulin pumps and blood glucose
meters*
www.accu-chek.co.uk

A Menarini Diagnostics
Tel: 01189 444 100
www.menarinidiag.co.uk
Blood glucose meters

Bayer
www.bayer.co.uk
*Pharmaceutical company
Manufactures blood glucose meters
and provides helpline*

Becton, Dickinson & Co
Tel: 01865 748844
www.bd.com
*Manufactures insulin pens, syringes
and needles and provides helpline*

British Heart Foundation (BHF)
Helpline: 0300 330 3311
www.bhf.org.uk
*Funds research, promotes education
and raises money to buy equipment
to treat people with heart disease.
For list of publications, posters and
videos, send s.a.e. Their helpline,
HeartstartUK, can arrange training in
emergency life-saving techniques for
lay people.*

British Parachute Association
5 Wharf Way
Glen Parva
Leicester LE2 9TF
Tel: 01162 785271
www.bpa.org.uk
*Governing body of sport parachuting.
Offers medical assessment on
suitability for parachuting to people
with medical disorders.*

British Hypertension Society
Tel: 020 8979 8300
www.bhsoc.org
*Charity providing services and advice
to healthcare professionals working
in the field of hypertension and
cardiovascular disease*

British Sub-Aqua Club
Telford's Quay
South Pier Road
Ellesmere Port
Cheshire CH65 4FL
Tel: 01513 506200
www.bsac.com
Governing body for sub-aqua sport.
Offers medical assessment for those
with medical disorders wanting to take
part in diving underwater.

Cobalt Systems Ltd
The Old Mill House
Mill Road, Reedham
Norwich, Norfolk, NR13 3TL
Tel: 01493 700172
Fax: 01493 701037
www.cobolt.co.uk
Supplier of products for the blind and
visually impaired

CP Pharmaceuticals
Now merged to form Wockhardt UK

Cygnus UK
Previously supplied Glucowatch, a
continuous blood sugar monitor. There
were a number of technical problems
and Glucowatch has been withdrawn.

Department of Health (DoH)
Produces and distributes literature
about public health. National Service
Framework for Diabetes can be
obtained from:
www. doh.gov.uk/en/Publicationsandstatistics/
Publications/PublicationPolicyandGuidance/
DH_4002951

Diabetes Research and Wellness Foundation
101–102 Northney Marina
Hayling Island
Hampshire PO11 0NH
Tel: 02392 637 808
www.drwf.org.uk
A diabetes support organisation based
in Washington DC, USA with a base
in the UK. Funds medical research;
its members receive newsletters with
personal stories and a question and
answer section.

Diabetes UK
10 Parkway
London NW1 7AA
Helpline: 020 7424 1030/1000
Careline: 0845 120 2960
Fax: 020 7424 1001
www.diabetes.org.uk
Provides advice and information on
diabetes; has local support groups

DiagnoSys Medical
Helpline: 0800 08 588 08
Distributors of blood glucose monitors and a range of other products via mail order

Diesetronic Medical Systems
This pump manufacturer has been taken over by the American giant Roche, who now supply insulin pumps under the name AccuCheks

Disability Alliance
Universal House
88–94 Wentworth Street
London E1 7SA
Tel: 020 7247 8776
Helpline: 020 7247 8763
www.disabilityalliance.org
Produces the Disability Rights Handbook. *Updated three times a year, it addresses every aspect of social services benefits for people with disabilities. Offers advice on benefits and training for other organisations and is involved with policy issues.*

GlaxoSmithKline
Tel: 020 8047 5000
Helpline: 0800 221441
www.gsk.co.uk
Manufactures drugs, provides information via helpline

The Guide Dogs for the Blind Association
Burghfield Common
Reading RG7 3YG
Tel: 0118 983 5555
www.guidedogs.org.uk
Provides guide dogs, mobility and other rehabilitation services that enable blind and partially sighted people to lead the fullest and most independent lives possible

Health Development Agency
Formerly the Health Education Authority and now taken over by NICE

Health Professionals Council
Park House
184 Kennington Park Road
London SE11 4BU
Tel: 020 7582 0866
Fax: 020 7820 9684
www.hpc-uk.org
Statutory regulator working to safeguard the health and well-being of people using the services of health professionals in the UK

Heart UK
7 North Road
Maidenhead SL6 1PE
Tel: 01628 628638
Helpline: 0845 450 5988
Fax: 01628 628698
www.heartuk.org.uk
The cholesterol charity that will help anyone at high risk of heart attack, but specialises in inherited conditions causing high cholesterol (familial hypercholesterolaemia)

HeartstartUK
see under British Heart Foundation

The Impotence Association
see under The Sexual Advice Association

Insulin Dependent Diabetes Trust
PO Box 294
Northampton NN1 4XS
Tel: 01604 622837
www.iddt.org
Trust set up to help and advise people having problems with human insulin. Collects insulin for distribution in developing countries. Also runs Sponsor a child scheme for a clinic in India.

Insulin-Pumpers UK
Website: www.insulin-pumpers.org.uk.
Offers information on the use of pumps and puts people in touch with each other. Advises on obtaining funding if pumps are not available via the NHS.

John Bell & Croyden
50–54 Wigmore Street
London W1U 2AU
Tel: 020 7935 5555
www.johnbellcroyden.co.uk
Dispensing pharmacy that can obtain medicines not manufactured in the UK, with appropriate named patient prescription and import licence

Juvenile Diabetes Research Foundation
19 Angel Gate
City Road
London EC1V 2PT
Tel: 020 7713 2030
www.jdrf.org.uk
Dedicated to funding research to find a cure for Type 1 diabetes. Provides information on the progress of research via leaflets, newsletters and open meetings.

LifeScan
Helpline: 0800 121200
www.lifescan.co.uk
Manufactures blood glucose monitoring systems and meters and offers advice

Eli Lilly Diabetes Care Division
Helpline: 0800 850777
General enquiries: 01256 315000
www.lilly.co.uk
Pharmaceutical company. Offers helpline to people with diabetes.

Medica Alarm
The Old Barn
Court Farm
Overstone
Northampton NN6 0AP
Tel: 01604 646200
Email: sales@medicalarm.co.uk

Medic-Alert Foundation
1 Bridge Wharf
156 Caledonian Road
London N1 9UU
Helpline: 0800 581420
www.medicalert.org.uk
*Offers a body-worn identification
system for people with hidden medical
conditions, and a selection of jewellery
with an internationally recognised
medical symbol. Has 24-hour
emergency telephone number.*

MediSense Britain
see under Abbotts Diabetes Care

**NICE The National Institute for
Health and Clinical Excellence**
(London office)
Midcity Place
71 High Holborn
London WC1V 6NA
Tel: 0845 003 7780
www.nice.org.uk

National Kidney Federation
The Point
Coach Road
Shireoaks
Worksop
S81 8BW
Helpline: 0845 601 0209
www.kidney.org.uk
*Provides information, campaigns for
improvement in care and supports
people through its network of local
groups*

Novartis
Helpline: 01276 698370
www.novartis.co.uk
Pharmaceutical company

Novo Nordisk
Helpline: 0845 600 5055
www.novonordisk.co.uk
*Manufactures injecting pens for
diabetes, growth hormone and HRT
injections*

Owen Mumford
Tel: 01993 812021
www.owenmumford.com
*Manufactures medical products for
people with diabetes*

Roche Diagnostics
Helpline: 0800 701000
www.roche-diagnostics.co.uk
*Manufactures blood glucose monitoring
system and insulin pumps under the
name AccuChek. Offers advice.*

The Royal National Institute of the Blind
105 Judd Street
London WC1H 9NE
Helpline: 0303 123 9999
Tel: 020 7388 1266
www.rnib.org.uk
Offers a range of information and advice on lifestyle changes and employment for people facing loss of sight. Also offers support and training in braille. Mail order catalogue of useful aids.

Sanafi-aventis
Tel: 01483 505 515
Fax: 020 7388 2034
www.sanafi-aventis.co.uk
Manufactures diabetes meters, offers advice

Servier Laboratories
Tel: 01753 662744
www.servier.co.uk
Manufactures diabetes meters, offers advice

Sexual Advice Association
Helpline: 020 7486 7262
www.sda.uk.net
Formerly the Sexual Dysfunction Association. Offers a listening ear and information on currently prescribed treatment and how sufferers should proceed to get best advice. Can advise on local specialists in erectile dysfunction.

Society of Chiropodists and Podiatrists
1 Fellmonger's Path
Tower Bridge Road
London SE1 3LY
Tel: 020 7234 8620
Fax: 0845 450 3721
www.feetforlife.org
Largest professional body representing over 8000 practising podiatrists. Offers foot health advice and information.

SOS Talisman
21 Grays Corner
Ley Street
Ilford IG2 7RQ
www.sostalisman.co.uk
Provides body-worn identification accessories for people with a range of hidden medical conditions

Stroke Association
240 City Road
London EC1V 2PR
Helpline: 0303 303 3100
www.stroke.org.uk
Funds research and provides information, specialising in stroke only

Sydney University's Glycaemic Index Research Service (SUGiRS)
Human Nutrition Unit Department of Biochemistry
G08 Sydney University
New South Wales 2006
Australia
Tel: 0061 2 9351 3757
Fax: 0061 2 9351 6022
www.glycemicindex.com
Commercial research and advisory service that measures GI values for foods, drinks and nutritional supplements. Provides advice to manufacturers to assist them in making low-GI products.

Takeda Pharmaceuticals
Tel: 01628 537900
Fax: 01628 526615
www.takeda.co.uk
Pharmaceutical manufacturers

Therasense
Customer Service line:
0800 138 5467
www.therasense.com
Manufactures blood glucose meters

Wockhardt UK
Tel: 01978 661261
Fax: 01978 660130
www.wockhardt.co.uk.
Committed to the production of porcine and bovine insulin

Index

Numbers in *italic* indicate pages with an illustration; those followed by italic *g* refer to glossary entries

acarbose (Glucobay®) 50, 56–7, 59, 275*g*
Acesulfane-K 275*g*
ACE inhibitor 132, 242
acetone 275g, 281*g*
acromegaly 16, 17
Actoplus Met® 50, 54, 59
Actos® *see* pioglitazone
Actrapid® *70*, 78, 92
acupuncture and diabetes 62
adrenaline 99, *101*, 166, 275*g*
AIDS 74
aircast ('Beckham Boot') 237
airport security and diabetic supplies 150
albumin 126, 218, 240, 241, 242, 275*g*, *see also* protein
alcohol and diabetes 98, 161, 173–4
  beneficial effects of 174
  and blood sugar 173–4
  guidelines 36–7, *37*, 40
  and hypos 161, 174–4, *270*
  in pregnancy 204
alpha cell 275g, 279*g*
alpha glucosidase inhibitor 50, 59, 276*g*
alprostadil (Caverject®) 191
alternative medicine and diabetes 63
Alzheimer's disease and diabetes 181
amitriptyline 243
amputation and diabetic gangrene 249–50
amyotrophy, diabetic 247, 278*g*
angina 248

angiography 276*g*
angioplasty 247, 276*g*
antibiotics 245
antigens 276*g*
antihistamines 163
Apidra® *70*, 76
apomorphine (Uprima®) 190
appetite, poor, and insulin 96
appetite suppressants and diabetes 45–6
arterial disease 247, 276*g*
arteries 247
arteriosclerosis 276*g*
aspart *70*, 76, 78–9, 92, 93, 156, 259
aspartame (Nutrasweet®) 31, 276*g*
asthma 68, 164
  asthma drugs and diabetes 14
atherosclerosis 232
athlete's foot 231
Attendance Allowance 180–1
Avandamet® 50, 53, 59
Avandia® *see* rosiglitazone
Aventis 76, 259

babies, large, and maternal diabetes 6, 13, 200, 201, 202, 210–11, 214
  and hypoglycaemia after birth 202, 211–12
  jaundiced 211
Balance (Diabetes UK magazine) 184, 228, 265
balanitis 22, 276*g*
Banting, Frederick 65, 255
basal bolus insulin regime *see under* insulin
BD Safe-Clip® 85
Bell's palsy 244

Benefits Agency 180
Best, Charles 65, 255
beta-blockers and diabetes 176, 276*g*
beta cell 4, 9, 276*g*
Betnovate® and diabetes 175
biguanides 50, 59, 146, 276*g*
Biostator 263
blindness and diabetes 216
blood circulation, poor 247
    see also feet
blood donation and diabetes 181
Blood Glucose Self-Monitoring
    Guidelines 141–3
blood glucose levels 4, 4, 13, 33–4,
    42, 53, 54, 58, 78–9, 92
    achieving control 29–30, 75,
    105ff, 257
    blood glucose and breast feeding
        206–7
    blood glucose, high 42, 52, 54, 58,
        114, 186, 198, 258
        and 'diabetic' foods 40
        effects on sex life 185
        effects of smoking on 177
        fertility 211
        potential for diabetic
            complications 58
        and vision *221*
        see hyperglycaemia
    blood glucose meters 51, 100,
        113–14, *116–17*, 118, 119,
        120, 121, 122, 123, 129, 276*g*
        for checking from arm 118, 123
        and travelling 149, 159
    blood glucose meters for the blind
        124
    control and complications in
        diabetes 215
    erratic levels and potency 186
    and exercise 48
    factors affecting glucose level 5,
        6–7, 51

glucose sensor 261
glucose testing: blood and urine
    tests compared 125–7
glucose tolerance test 113, 127,
    279*g*
glucose in urine 3, 124, 125, 126
and heart disease 248–51
and illness 58
measurements *112*
and missed injections 78–9
monitoring 10, 98, 105, 111–14,
    261, 276*g*
    non-invasive 261
    shift work 158
    sticks 110, 276*g*
    sticks, storage of 113
normal blood glucose levels 109,
    111
stress 165–6
and tablets 53, 57, 58
tests for blood glucose levels 96,
    104, 108ff
testing and travel 155–7
transition from tablets to insulin 58
see also haemoglobin, glycosylated
    (HbA$_{1c}$), pregnancy
blood pressure and diabetes 251–2
low blood pressure 252
high blood pressure 133, 252
and kidney problems 251
blood sugar *see* blood glucose
blood sugar, low *see* hypoglycaemia
blood supply, poor (ischaemia) 237
blood testing 113–14
blood testing strips 110, 113–14,
    116–17, 119, 121, 123, 141–2
    cost of 110, 112, 126
    availability on prescription
        114, 120, 124
    and travel 149, 155
    use of 118
at home 118–20, 122

home and hospital compared
120–1
storage 113
testing from arm 123
at 3 a.m. 104, 130
using laser 123–4
and visual impairment 124
brain damage and diabetes 253
haemorrhage and diabetes 252
breathalyser tests and diabetes 172
British Diabetic Association (now
Diabetes UK) 264
British Hypertension Society 251
British Parachute Association 146
British Sub-Aqua Club 145
bronchodilators 177
bunions 231

Caesarean section 202, 211, 213–4
calories and content in foods 29, 31,
32–3, 40, 276g
Candida (thrush) 21, 195–6
cannabinoid blocker 258–9
CAPD (chronic ambulatory
peritoneal dialysis) 241
carbohydrates 35, 36, 41, 42, 58,
111, 146 passim, 180, 270,
275g, 276g, 277g, 279g, 284g
alcohol and 37, 173–4
alpha glucosidase inhibitor and 50
acarbose and 54
breastfeeding 206
content of food 32–3
diet and 90, 93, 98
emergency foods and 272
food labelling 32
and glycaemic index (GI) 38, 92, 98
and healthy eating 39
and hypoglycaemia 100, 103, 191
insulin and 74, 90, 95, 148-9
travel, diabetes and carbohydrates
149, 150, 157

carpal tunnel syndrome 245
cataract 227, 276g
and diabetes 22, 225
Caverject® (alprostadil) 191
Cell Robotics 123
CEMACH *see* Confidential Enquiry
into Maternal and Child Health
Charcot process (feet) 237, 277g
children
and diabetes 9
and glucagon 103, 104
and obesity 9–10, 11
Type 1 diabetes 12
Type 2 11–12
Chiropodists and Podiatrists, Society
of 230
chiropody *see* podiatry
cholesterol 11, 12, 39, 44, 49, 154,
250
types of 49
and brain haemorrhage 252
cholesterol lowering tablets 219
and contraceptive pill 192
HDL 49, 259
heart disease 133, 248, 249
LDL 49
and pregnancy 205
and rimonabant 259
chronic ambulatory peritoneal
dialysis (CAPD) 241
Cialis® 189–90
Citizen's Advice Bureau 160, 161
CITR 257
claudication, intermittent 232
Cobolt Systems Ltd 124
Coca-Cola 208
coma 277g
complementary therapies and
diabetes 63
complications arising from diabetes
Chapter 8
genetic component 219

Confidential Enquiry into Maternal and Child Health (CEMACH) 200, 205, 276*g*
contact lenses and diabetes 225
contraception 186, 192
contraceptive pill 14, 177, 192–3
control *see* blood glucose
corn (feet) and remedies 230, 232, 234, *239*
counselling and impotence 191
cough medicines and diabetes 176, 177
creatinine 131, 154
Cushing's disease/syndrome 15, 16
Cygnus Inc. 121
cystic fibrosis 16
cystitis 240, 241, 277*g*

DAFNE programme (for diabetics) 25, 148, 277*g*
Delivery Strategy (for diabetes) 138, 139
dental work and diabetes 167
depression 164, 165, 186, 253
    and difficulty of achieving good control 165
    rimonabant and 259
DESMOND programme (Diabetes Education Self Management Ongoing and Newly Diagnosed) 25, 26, 27, 28, 164–7, 253, 277*g*
detemir (Levemir®) 76, 77, 78, 259, 277*g*
Dextro-Energy tablets 208, *271, 272*
Diabetic amyotrophy 247, 278*g*
diabetes:
    and abortion 198
    acupuncture and 62
    alternative/complementary medicine and 63
    and Disability Discrimination Act 160, 161
    appetite suppressants and 46
    asthma drugs and 14

blood glucose control and 105, 115
blurred vision and 22
and breastfeeding 206
brittle diabetes 276*g*
causes of diabetes 7ff
CENACH and 200
in children 7, 9
complications in 2, 69, Chapter 8
        genetic component 219
contraception 192ff
and congenital abnormalities 200, 201, 205, 210
        Type 1 and 2 *11*
control of 107, 109–11, 129, 220, *221*, 240
control by diet 29, 30ff
defined 1ff
and dental work 167
depression and 164–5
diabetes insipidus 6, 277*g*
diabetes mellitus 6, 277*g*
diet and 24, 27ff, 43, 129
differences between Type 1 and Type 2 5–6, *11–12*
and driving 159
and eating out 148
educational programmes 25ff
ethnicity and 17–18, 30, 35, 36
excess thirst and 20
and fasting 149
and feet 229ff
and fertility 198
gestational diabetes *see* under pregnancy
guidelines for healthy eating *39–40*
hay fever, allergies and 163
heart attacks and 16, 23, 80
herbal remedies and 63
hospital operations and 166
in India 9
inheritance/genetic component 7, 8, 194, 202–3

and insulin production 4ff
insulin and 28, 33–4, Chapter 3
and keep fit 146–7
lipoatrophic diabetes 220, 281*g*
long-term complications of, 183
    Chapter 8, 277*g*
monitoring Chapter 4
national frameworks for diabetes
    25
obesity and 8, 28
other illnesses and 12–13, 162ff
other medical conditions inducing
    diabetes 12, 16
out of control diabetes 52
pancreatic transplants 281
pneumonia and 16
poor control 69, 125, 126, 129,
    143, 147, 175, 200, 201, 203,
    209, 217, 225, 252
        and blood flow 249
        and heart disease 248, 249
        and illnesses 162, 163–4
possible prevention of 255
and pregnancy *see under* pregnancy
relaxation techniques and 62
research on 255
self-monitoring of diabetes 105
and sleep 160
and sport 145–7
stress and 12, 63, 110, 165
and sunbathing 152
symptoms of 20ff
tablets prescribed 9, 18, 50ff, 107
temporary diabetes 12
transplantation of islets of
    Langerhans 257
and travel sickness tablets 150
travel abroad 149ff
treatment without insulin Chapter
    2
types of, defined 5ff
US study on *11*–12, 13

and vaccination 153
vaccination against 255
and vaginal itching 21
weight and 97, 258–9
weight loss and 20–1
see also alcohol, blood sugar,
    Diabetes UK, diet, hypoglycaemia
    (hypos), insulin, pancreas,
    pregnancy, Chapter 11
    (Emergencies)
diabetes: Type 1 (insulin dependent
    diabetes, IDD, juvenile-onset
    diabetes) 1, 5–6, 65, 280*g*, 284*g*
complications 218
diagnosis 22
and high density lipoprotein 49
inheritance and 16, 19
and insulin production 5
islets of Langerhans transplant 257
lipoatrophic diabetes 220
monitoring *142*
treatment of 65
see also pregnancy
diabetes: Type 2 (non-insulin
    dependent diabetes, NIDD) 1–2,
    6, 9, 26, 27, 44–5, 50, 65, 282*g*,
    284*g*
blood glucose self-monitoring
    guidelines 141–3
blood glucose testing 121
children and 10, *11*–12
complications 2, 218, 226
control of 54, 107–8, 257
diagnosis of 1–2, 22–3, 24
diet and 24, 34ff, 43, 217
epidemic of 13
exercise 13, 48–50
and glandular disorders 16
glitazones as treatment 55
HDL and 49
and haemoglobin, glycosylated
    (HbA$_{1c}$) 107

diabetes: Type 2 (*cont'd*)
  heart disease and stroke *11*, 133,
    250
  hypoglycaemia ('hypo') 104–5
  islets of Langerhans transplant 257
  and inheritance 16–17, 18, 19–20,
    202
  and insulin production 5
  insulin injections *11*, 43, 50
  insulin resistance 6, 28, 55
  life expectancy 219
  metformin and 53
  monitoring of 108, 110–11, 141–3
  obesity and 28, 43, 50
  poor control 50, 54, 113
  prospects with 108
  sport and 145–7
  swimming 145–6
  tablets, use of 1, 24, 33–4, 43,
    104–5, 121
  testing, need for 108–9
  tight control, need for 107
  treatment of Chapter 2, 54, 62
  type MODY (Maturity-Onset
    Diabetes of the Young) 18, 19, 202
  urine testing and 126
  in USA 9
  see also blood sugar, exercise,
    insulin, pregnancy
diabetes clinic 35, 105, 115, 130,
    131, 134, 232, 240, 241, 264
diabetes education 24ff
Diabetes Education Self Management
    Ongoing and Newly Diagnosed
    see DESMOND programme
Diabetic Foot Team 230, 237
Diabetes for beginners (Diabetes UK
    publication) 265
Diabetes UK Islet Transplantation
    Consortium 257
Diabetes National Service Framework
    (NSF) 26, 107, 138ff, 222

diabetes specialist nurse 45, 93, 97,
    103, 114, 115, 134, *136*
Diabetes UK (organisation) 128, 131,
    153, 161, 184, 264–6
  Diabetes UK Careline 33, 35, 155,
    179–80, 265
  booklets and factsheets 34, 133,
    147, 265
  Care Support team 267
  and driving 168, 170
  holidays, provision of 265–6
  insurance provision 152, 170,
    265
  Insurance Services 265–6
  Local Support Groups 25, 27, *136*,
    253, 254, 265
  and 'missing millions' 7
  pregnancy magazine 202
  provision of treatment identity
    cards and other documents 150,
    151
  research and fundraising 67, 254,
    255
  on sport 147
  website 35, 255
  work issues 155, 168
  see also Balance, DAFNE, DESMOND,
    X-PERT
diabetic coma 278*g*
diabetic foods (marketing ploy) 31,
    40, 45, 278*g*
dialysis 240–1, 256
diarrhoea, diabetic 52, 53, 54, 98,
    245–6, 278*g*
diet and diabetes 8, 27ff, 38, 43,
    180
  guidelines on balanced diet 33, 35,
    39–40
  and hypoglycaemia 43
  and insulin 90ff
  and potential complications 217
  and weight gain 29, 34

dietary fibre 278*g*, 285*g*
dietitian 33, 34–5, 38, 40, 42, 45, 90, 90, 96
  State Registered Dietitian 34, 35
digital retinal photography 222–3
Disability Alliance 180
Disability Discrimination Act 160, 161, 170
Disability Living Allowance 179
diuretics 14, 175–6, 278*g*, 285*g*
dizziness 52, 100, 252
DPP-4 (dipeptyl peptidase 4) inhibitors 258
DREAM Study 13
driving and diabetes 159, *168*, 170–1, *270*, *271*
driving licences, PCV, HGV and LGV and diabetes 168, 171–2
Driving and Vehicle Licensing Agency (DVLA) 168–9, 170
DVT 192

ear piercing *144*, 182
eating plan 90–2
Edmonton Protocol 257
educational programmes for diabetes 25ff
electric blankets and diabetes 181, *235*
electrolysis *144*, 184
emergencies Chapter 11
epidural 278*g*
epilepsy 102
erectile dysfunction 187, 186ff, 278*g*, 280*g*
  and counselling 191
  see also apomorphine, Cialis®, Viagra®
European Health Insurance Card (EHIC) 150, 155
Exenatide® 61
exercise and diabetes 47–9, 98, 247

Exubera® (inhaled insulin) 68, 69, 259
eyes and diabetes 22, 58, 108, *221*ff
  age-related changes in sight 228
  checks 221–2
  eye damage *see* retinopathy
  digital retinal photography 222–3
  effects of diabetes on 223
  laser treatment of 170, 226, 227
  see also retina, retinopathy, vision

fasting and diabetes 148–9
fats 39, 90, 98, 98
feet and diabetes 229ff, 244
  damage to foot 152
  effects of diabetes 232ff
  effects of winter/cold 233, *234–5*
  'feet facts' *234*
Foot Care Rules 236, 237, *238–9*
  numbness 236
  swelling of 237
  toenails 229, 231, *238*, *239*
  ulcers on feet 152, 182, 218, 236
  walking barefoot 233, *239*
fertility and diabetes 198–9
fibre *see* dietary fibre
finger pricking, for blood tests 118–9, 123–4
first aid and feet *239*
fludrocortisone 252
fluid retention 55, 54
folic acid 205–6, 209, 210
food labels *32–3*
  traffic light system 33
foods, emergency *272*
food plan 41–2, 90–2
  see also guidelines on balanced diet
foot spa and diabetes 184
FreeStyle® Freedom and FreeStyle Mini 123
fructose 31
fructosamine 278*g*
  test 128–9

fruit juice and blood glucose 42
fungicide 184, 231

gabapentin 240
gangrene 177, 216, 230, 232, 249,
    278*g*
gastroparesis 246, 278*g*
GI *see* glycaemic index
ginseng 64
glandular disorders 16
glargine (Lantus®) 71, 76, 77, 259,
    277g, 279*g*
glasses and diabetes *221*, 221
glaucoma and diabetes 227, 279*g*
GlaxoSmithKline (GSK) 54
glibenclamide 50, 54, 59, 104
gliclazide 14, 48, 50, 50, 53, 54–5,
    54, 58, 130
    possible side effects 52, 54, 104
glimepiride 50, 59
gliptins *see* DPP-4 inhibitors
glipizide 50, 59
gliquidone 59
glitazone 55, 54, 104, 258, 279*g*
glucagon 2, 3–4, 14, 61, 103–4,
    150–3
    effects of ingestion 103
    and GLP-1 259
GLP-1 (glucagon-like peptide) 259,
    258, 279*g*
Glucobay® (acarbose) 50, 54–6
glucogel (Hypostop®) 150, 208, *271*
Glucophage® *see* metformin
glucose 3, 4, 20–1, 103, 276g, 279g,
    see also blood glucose
GlucoWatch® 121–2
glycaemic index (GI) 38, 91, 92, 93,
    94
    glycaemic control 69
glycogen 3, 279*g*
glycosylated haemoglobin *see*
    haemoglobin A$_{1c}$

GP (General Practitioner)
    and diabetes 5, 21, 25, 26, 85,
        118, 151
    diabetic clinics 35, 131, 133, 134
    and blood glucose testing 110, 111,
        113, 120, 121, 129
    and form for exemption from
        prescription charges 179
    and payment for targets *140*
    and retinal screening 224
    and treating diabetes 133, 134
growth hormone treatment 177
guidelines on healthy eating/
    balanced diet 33, 35, *39–40*, 41,
        107–80
gustatory sweating 244

haemochromatosis (iron overload) 16
haemodialysis 241
haemoglobin, glycosylated (HbA$_{1c}$)
    57, 69, 107, 120, 126, 127–8,
        216, 219
    achieving normal levels 104–5
    and eyes 226
    and GLP-1 259
    introduction of 105
    and pregnancy 199, 200, 209,
        210, 213
    purpose of test 127–8
    and rimonabant 259
    testing 127–8, 129, *140, 141*
hay fever 163
HbA$_{1c}$ *see* haemoglobin, glycosylated
Health Professions Council 230
Health, Department of 138
healthcare team *135*
heart attacks and diabetes 16, 23,
        133, 192
    and insulin 80
    and Viagra® 190
heart disease 108, 215, 247, 277*g*
    and Type 2 diabetes 219

heart failure 175
high blood pressure 219, 247
holidays and diabetes 149ff
   checklist 149–50, 154–5
honeymoon period (insulin) 279*g*
hormones 2, 14, 15, 271g, 279*g*
   and diabetes 14ff
   and erectile dysfunction 191
hormone replacement therapy (HRT)
   177, 196
hospital operations 166
hot water bottles and diabetes 182,
   235, 236, 239
Humalog® *see* lispro
Humulin S *70*, 92, M3 *72*
hydramnios 211–2, 279*g*
hyperglycaemia (high blood glucose)
   274, 280*g*
hypoglycaemia ('hypo') (low blood
   glucose) 2, 14, 100ff, 109,
   110, 113, *137*, 138, *142, 143,*
   180–1, 269–71, 280*g*
   dealing with 100–1
   signs of 100, *101*, 273
   and adrenaline production 100
   and alcohol 161, 173–4
   arm samples and 123
   babies, newborn and 7, 202, 204,
      211–4, 213
   beta-blockers and 176, 276g,
      279g, 280*g*
   and breastfeeding 206
   brain damage, possibility of 253
   causes of 100
   dentistry 167
   diet and 30, 43, 96, 98, 166
   and dizziness 52
   and drinking 173–4
   driving and 159, 168, 170–4
   exercise and 48, 49
   and fasting 149
   and fits 102

foreign travel 155, *157*
glucagon 103
   and gliclazide 52, 54
glycaemic index 92, 93
   and habituation to varying levels of
      blood glucose 114
   and human insulin 67
   and other illnesses 162, 163
   informing work colleagues 159–60
   and insulin analogues 76
   insulin regimes 74, 76, 78, 97
   isophane insulin *71*, 76
   night time 74, 76, 93, *94*, 104, 130
   possibility of memory loss 253
   pregnancy 202, 208
   risks of 102, *143*
   sex and 191
   and shifting meal times 96
   and sport 145, 146, 152
   sunbathing 152, 182
   symptoms of/warning signs 99,
      102, 105
   tablets and 104–5
   and timing of insulin dose 100
   testing blood sugar and 109, 123
   and travelling through time zones
      155
   treatment of 100
   and use of human insulin 67
   vomiting 103
   warning signs 67, 99, 102, 105,
      159, 171, 176, 226, *270, 271*
   warning signals and beta-blockers
      276*g*
   and workmates 159–60
   work patterns 159
hypoglycaemic attacks 105
   and pregnancy 208
hypoglycaemic coma 105, *273*
Hypoguard Ltd 154
Hypostop® (Glucogel) 150, *271*
Hypurin, porcine and bovine *70*

ice-cream 45–6
identification bracelet/necklace/card
    144, 149
illness and blood glucose levels 58
insulin/tablet use and hypos 104–5
immunosuppressive therapy 257
impotence *see* erectile dysfunction
Improvement, Expansion and Reform:
    the next three years (Diabetes NSF
    strategy document) 139
indigestion tablets and diabetes 175
infertility 198–9
inhalers 261
inheritance and diabetes 7, 16ff
injector 85, 280*g*
InnoLet® *83*, 87, 280*g*
Insuman Rapid *70*
Insulatard 78
insulin 2, 4, 7, 21, 43, 146, *270*
    age and insulin reduction 82
    analogues 76
    and air travel 150–3
    allergic reactions 74
    basal bolus regimen *71*, 75, 84, 85,
        93, 96, *142*, 155–6, 158, 159,
        160, *168*
    terms defined 74, 77
    beef based (bovine) 66, *70*, *71*, 153
    biosynthetic 259
    body's need for 3ff
    brain damage, possibility of 102,
        103
    clear insulin 66, *70*, *71*, 76, 277*g*
    cloudy insulin *71*, 277*g*
    delivery, developments in 259ff
    and depression 103
    and diabetes 4ff
    diet and insulin 90ff, 97–98
    discovery of insulin 65, 215, 255
    dosage 80
    effectiveness of different methods of
        insulin provision 259–0

and exercise 48, 49, 90
fast-acting 76
and festive eating 94
forgetting injections 78
and glucagon 103
heart attacks and 80
holiday/travel checklist 149–50,
    154–5
human insulin 66, 67, 68, 74, 153,
    259, 268, 279*g*
and illnesses 162
inhaled insulin 66, 68–9, 259
insulin levels and menstrual cycle
    114–15
insulin production system 4
insulin reactions and potential for
    brain damage 1023
insulin regimes 75–6, 78, 95, 96
insulin resistance 6, 8, 28–9, 43,
    50, 54, 55, 199, 279g, 280*g*
insulin treatment 54, 58–1,
    Chapter 3
intermediate insulin 67, *71*, 74,
    75, 99, 104, 158, 280g, 281*g*
isophane *70*, 76, 99, 280*g*
lente insulin *72*, 281*g*
and long stays abroad 153ff
and meals 92
multiple injection regime 84, 85
nasal sprays 259
need for injection 66, 68
and oral contraceptives 115
pork based (porcine) 66, 67–8, *70*,
    71, *72*, 74, 153, 283*g*
seasonal variations in usage 82
short-acting 283*g*
and snacks 93, 94–5
soluble *70*, 99
storage of 89
and suicide attempts/risk 103, 253
testing 108–9
and time zones 155–6, *157*

timing of injections 74, 77, 80,
  82ff, 92–4, 95
and travel 157
types of 66ff, 70–1, 74, 74, 76–9,
  78, 276g, 277g, 277g, 281g,
  280g
U40 insulin 153, 285g
U100 insulin 153, 285g
and use of tablets 54, 58, 61
see also blood sugar testing,
  pancreas, insulin pens, injectors,
  individual brand names, Chapter
  11 (Emergencies)
Insulin Dependent Diabetes Trust
  (IDDT) 268–9
insulin injecting 43, 58, 66, 82ff, 93,
  96, 130, 259
  devices 61
  disposal of devices 85
  injectors 85ff
  needles 86
  reuse 85
  selection of 86
  syringes 82, 85–6, 87, 88, 149
  visual impairment and selection of
    82, 87
insulin pens 66, 67, 73, 74, 77,
  82–3, 83, 85, 148, 159, 280g
insulin pump 122, 213, 261–3
Insulin-Pumpers 267
insulin reaction/insulin shock see
  hypoglycaemia
insulin user's identification card 150
insurance and diabetes 170
intradermal injections 280g
intramuscular injection 280g
intravenous glucose sensor 261
iron overload (haemochromatosis) 16
irritable bowel syndrome 246
ischaemia 237
Islet Transplantation Consortium
  (Diabetes UK) 257

islets of Langerhans 2, 280g
  transplant of 256–
isophane see under insulin
IUD (intrauterine contraceptive
  device) 195

Jewish Diabetic Association 36
John Bell & Croyden 154
joule 29, 280g
Juvenile Diabetes Research
  Foundation (JDRF) 267–8

keep fit 146–7
ketoacidosis 105, 281g
ketones 21, 116, 281g
  and breathalysers 172
  in urine 125, 126
ketonuria 281g
kidney problems 251
  damage 126, 131, 240
  disease 126, 192, 240ff
  failure 132, 218, 240
  transplants 241, 256
  see also nephropathy, National
    Kidney Federation

lancet, use of 85, 118, 119, 123
Lantus® see glargine
laser treatment of eyes 224, 226,
  281g
  and driving 170
  scarring 227
Lasette 123–4
Lawrence, R D 264
legs and diabetes 246, 247
Levemir® see detemin
Levitra® 190
LifeScan (company) 123
Lilly (firm) 83, 257, 259
Lion Alcolmeter 172
Lions International 27
lipohypertrophy 69, 281g

lipoprotein: low density (LDL) and
high density (HDL) 49, 259
Liraglutide® 257–9
lispro (Humalog®) *70, 73,* 76, 78,
80, 92, 93, 156, 259
liver 3–4
London Marathon 147
loperamide 246
Lucozade 100, 145, 162, 191, 208,
270, 271, 272
lungs and use of inhaled insulin 68,
259

malaria 153
Maturity-Onset Diabetes of the Young
(MODY) *see* Diabetes Type 2
MedicAlarm 181
Medic-Alert 183
medical identity discs and bracelets
144, 150, 183
Medical Research Council 254
medical waste, disposal of 85
Mendosa, David 36
menopause 193, 196
metabolic
control 55
rate 281*g*
syndrome *11,* 259, 281*g*
metabolism 281*g*
meters, blood sugar *see under* blood
glucose
metformin tablets (Glucophage®)
50, 53, 54, 55, 54, 54, 59, 258,
276g, 281g, 283*g*
health benefits of 53
intolerance to 54, 130
side effects 52, 53, 54, 54, 104
starting use of 8
tablet types 50
and Type 2 diabetes 13, 50, 53
US study on 13
metoclopramide 246

MHI-500 85
microalbuminuria 126, 131–2, 154,
240, 242, 281*g*
microaneurysms 226, 281*g*
micromole, defined 281*g*
millimole, defined 111–12, 282*g*
Minimed Medtronic (device) 122,
261
Mixtard *72,* 75, 115
MODY (Maturity-Onset Diabetes of
the Young) *see* Diabetes Type 2
motor insurance 170

nateglinide (Starlix®) 50, 54, 54, *59,*
282*g*
national framework for diabetes 25
National Institute for Clinical
Excellence *see* NICE
National Kidney Federation (NKF)
268
National Service Framework (NSF)
see Diabetes National Service
Framework
Nauru islanders and diabetes 18
nausea 52, 54
Navidrex® 176
needles
disposal of *137*
selection of 86
nephropathy, diabetic 216, 217, 218,
241, 278g, 282*g*
PKC and 258
nerve damage 243–5
see also amyotrophy, neuropathy,
neuritis
neuritis 243
facial 244
neuropathy, 183, 216, 217, 218,
243, 244, 258, 278g, 282*g*
and acupuncture 62
autonomic neuropathy 245, 246,
252, 276g, 278*g*

and feet 152, 184, 216, 229, 230, 232–3, 236, 237, 244, 277*g*
and gangrene 278*g*
and hands 245
and legs 246
pain relief and 243
peripheral 282*g*
PKC and 258
and sexual problems 187, 191
NHS prescriptions – how to get them free 179
NHS 27, 139, 189, 283*g*
NICE (National Institute for Clinical Excellence UK medical watchdog) 54, 68–9, 282g, 283*g*
nicotine and patches 177–8
nitrate drugs and Viagra® 190
Novo Nordisk 82, *83*, 87, 259, 259, 259
NovoNorm® 149
NovoRapid® *see* aspart
Nutech International 124
Nutrasweet® (aspartame) 31, 276*g*
nutritional information *32, 33 see also* diet and diabetes

obesity 1, 6
in children 9–10
and diabetes 8, 9, 43
central obesity 29, 30, 40
and heart disease 248
oedema 240
Omega 3 fat *39*
OneTouch® Ultra 123
OptiClik® Pen *83*
oral hypoglycaemic agents (OHA) 69
orlistat (Xenical®) 46, 98, 282g, 285*g*
orthotist 236
osteoporosis 197
Owen Mumford (Medical Shop) *83*, 85, 118

pancreas 2, 3, 14, 54, 282*g*
artificial 261, 263
cancer of 16
diseases of 16
and glucagon production 103
and insulin production 28, 50, 82, 85, 93, 259
pancreatic transplantation 256
pancreatitis 15–16
papaverine 191
parachuting (sport) and diabetes 146
penile implant 191
penis and diabetes 21
PenMate® 82
peripheral neuropathy 282*g*
Pfizer 259
phimosis 21, 282*g*
photocoagulation 282g, *see also* laser treatment
photography, digital retinal 222–3
Pima (native Americans) and diabetes 17, 18
pioglitazone (Actos®) 50, 55–6, 59, 282g, 282*g*
PKC (protein kinase C) inhibitors 258, 282*g*
plasma 128
pneumonia 16
podiatrist 229, 230, 231–2, *238*, 250
podiatry 229ff, 236
polydipsia 283*g*
polyuria 283*g*
postural hypotension 252
practice nurses 26, 35, 77, 108, 114, 129, 131, 132, 133, *136*, 164, *270*
and retinal screening 224
and treating diabetes patients 133, 134
prandial glucose regulators 50, 54, 59, 283*g*
Prandin® *see* repaglinide

prediabetes 13–14, 16
prednisolone 14
pre-eclampsia 283*g*
pregabalin 243
pregnancy and diabetes 6–7, 12,
    44–5, 115, *143*, 192, 198,
    Chapter 7
  and blood glucose levels 200–1,
    202–3, 208
  complications arising from 200–1,
    209ff
  and congenital abnormality 200–1,
    205, 209–200
  gestational diabetes 6–7, 13, 44,
    200, 208, 278*g*
  hydramnios 211–12
  hypoglycaemic attacks 208
  toxaemia 211
  termination 198, 210, 211
prescription charges 179ff
Primary Care 133
  Trusts 111, 179
  clinics 132
protein kinase C (PKC) inhibitors 258
protein 4, 20, *32*, 42, 49, 66, 68, 90,
    240, 241, 242, 283*g*
  cholesterol and 49
  in diet *32*, 42, 90, 98
  genetic engineering and insulin
    production 66, 68
  in urine 126, 131
  see also albumin
proteinuria 283*g*
pruritus vulvae 21, 184, 283*g*
pyelonephritis 240, 241, 283*g*

Quorn 98, 98

Ramadam 148–9
Reductil® (sibutramine) 46
relaxation techniques and diabetes
    62

renal glycosuria 124, 127
renal replacement therapy 240–1
renal threshold 113, 124, 126, 127,
    283*g*
repaglinide (Prandin®) 50, 54, 59,
    149, 283*g*
residential homes and diabetes
    183
respiratory distress syndrome (RDS)
    211, 214
retina 22, 283*g*
retinal screening 155, 283g,
    photography 218
retinopathy, diabetic 22, 138, 216,
    217, 278g, 283*g*
  defined 224
  and blindness 224–5
  contact lenses 225
  and eye checks 221–2
  and microaneurysms 226, 281*g*
  national screening 224
  PKC and 258
  proliferative retinopathy 227
  and short sightedness *221*
rheumatoid arthritis 14
rimonabant (Accomplia®) 45–6
rosiglitazone (Avandamet®,
    Avandia®) 13–14, 50, 54–7, 59,
    154, 283g,
  side effects 54–7
roughage 283*g*
Royal National Institute of the Blind
    (RNIB) 228

saccharine 31, 283*g*
salt in diet *39*, 251
Sanofi-Aventis *83*
saunas 182
Scotchcast 236
Scottish Inter-collegiate Guidelines
    Network (SIGN) 107
self-help groups Chapter 10

Self-Monitoring Guidelines, Blood Glucose *141–3*
SensoCard® Plus Meter 124
sex and hypoglycaemia 191
sexual function and diabetes Chapter 8
  and hypos 191
  loss of sexual interest 186, *186*
  see also erectile dysfunction
Shapiro, James 257
Sharps bin 85
shingles 244
shoes and diabetes 229, 232, *235, 234, 238*
short sightedness *221*
SI Units (Système International d'Unites) 111
sibutramine (Reductil®) 46
SIGN (Scottish Inter-collegiate Guidelines Network) 107
simvastatin *39*
skiing, winter sports and diabetes 146, 152
skin irritation 184
skin layers 87
'sliding scale' of insulin, after operations 166
smoking and diabetes 179–9, 220, 248, 250
  blood glucose monitoring *141*
  and Exubera 68
  health risks of 177, *177*, 192, 220, *239*, 247, 249
  and pregnancy 203–4
  and poor circulation 232
  quitting 177–8, 249
  and risk of gangrene 230, 232, 250
  and weight 177, *177*
Snellen Chart 284g, *285g*
Social Security benefits and diabetes 179

socks and diabetes 231
sorbitol, 31, 278g, 284*g*
SOS/Talisman 183–4
Special Care Baby Unit 211, 214
spina bifida 209, 210
sport and diabetes 145–7
  and hypos 145, 146
SQ-PEN 85
Standards of Care (for diabetes) 138
Starlix® *see* nateglinide
statin 252
sterilisation 194
steroids 110, 164, 177, 256, 284*g*
  and diabetes 175
  inducing diabetes 14–15
  and pregnancy 211, 214
stress 5, 12, 16, 28, 63, 110, 165–7, 186, 276*g*
strokes 216
  and diabetes 108, 134, 192, 196, 219, 250, 252
  and HRT 196
  and impotence 189
subcutaneous injection 284*g*
sucrose 284*g*
sugar 39, 40, 54
sulphonylurea group 48, 50, 54, *54*, *59*, 146, 149, 284*g*
  and alcohol 174
  and pregnancy 204
sunbathing, sunbeds and diabetes 152, 182
sweeteners, artificial 31, *32*, 40–1, 42
swimming and diabetes 145–6
symptoms of diabetes *see* diabetes
syringes *see* under insulin injecting

tablets for diabetes 50ff, 90, 104–5, 126, 130, 219–20, 269–70
  and blood sugar monitoring 112–3
  and drinking 173, 174

and driving 168, 171
and illness 58
and pregnancy 203
minimum and maximum doses
57–9
and transition to insulin 54, 58,
61, 173
testosterone 191
thiazide group of tablets 176, 177
thiazolidinediones 50, 59, 284*g*
thirst and diabetes 20
Thompson, Leonard 65
thrombosis 284*g*
thrush (Candida) 21, 195–6
thyrotoxicosis/hyperthyrodism 15,
16
tissue markers 284*g*
toenails and diabetes 229, 231, *238,
239*
ingrowing 229, 231
Torah 36
Toronto University, Physiology
Department 65
toxaemia 211, 284*g*
transplantation 256–8
travel and diabetes 149ff
travel insurance 152
travel sickness tablets and diabetes
150
triglycerides 259
triple oral therapy (in diabetes) 54
triple test (in pregnancy) 210
troglitazone 55
twin studies and diabetes 19–20
Type 1 diabetes *see* diabetes, Type 1
Type 2 diabetes *see* diabetes, Type 2

UK Prospective Diabetes Study
(UKPDS) 53, 107, 108, 132, 216,
220, 251
UK 54, 54, 107
Uprima® (apomorphine) 190

urine 4, 20, 21, 124–5
glucose in 21, 240
laboratory urine tests 127, 285*g*
protein in *see* albumin,
microalbuminuria
testing sticks 132
urine test 22, 54, 105, 112, 113,
121, 124, 125, *141, 143,* 240
USA and diabetes 9, 18

vaccination and diabetes 153
vacuum therapy 191
vagina and diabetes 21
vasectomy 193–4
Velosulin® *70*
venous thrombosis/deep vein
thrombosis/DVT 192
Ventolin® 177
vertigo and diabetes 182–3
Viagra® 189, 190, 191
and nitrate drugs 190
vidaglyptin 258
virus 285
vision, blurred, as symptom of
diabetes 22
visual acuity 285*g*
visual fields test 170
visual impairment and use of devices
89, 124, 228
visual problems and diabetes 170, 22,
225 *see also* eyes and diabetes
vomiting 103, 105, 150, 162, 246,
259, *271, 272,* 278g, 281*g*

water tablets *see* diuretics
weight control 40, 44, 45
weight gain 29, 34, 55, 97–8
weight loss 44–6, 50, 98–99, 258
weight loss as symptom of diabetes
20–1
Weight Watchers 47
Wellcome Trust 254

Wells, H G 264
What care to expect from your healthcare team (Diabetes UK guide) 108, *135–8*
What diabetes care to expect (Diabetes UK booklet) 132, 133
work and diabetes 158–61
  irregular hours 158–9

shift work 158
Work and Pensions, Department of 180
Workforce Development Confederation 139

Xenical® *see* orlistat
X-PERT 27

Become a member of Diabetes UK today

• •

Join Diabetes UK today to benefit from our bi-monthly members magazine, *Balance*, a network of support groups across the UK and confidential information and support from our Careline

To join today visit www.diabetes.org.uk/join

Or call 0800 138 5605

Please get in touch with us

Diabetes UK Careline is here to help. Call **0845 120 2960** for support and information. (Calls cost no more than 4p per minute, calls from mobiles usually cost more)

• •

The charity for people with diabetes
www.diabetes.org.uk
Registered charity no. 215199

009A01026

Have you found **Type 2 Diabetes: Answers at your fingertips** useful and practical? If so, you may be interested in other books from Class Publishing.

TYPE 2 DIABETES IN ADULTS OF ALL AGES

Dr Charles Fox and Dr Ragnar Hanas £19.99

This practical, easy-to-read book tells you everything you need to know about your diabetes. Bestselling authors Charles Fox and Ragnar Hanas have produced a comprehensive, no-nonsense manual that shows you, step by step, how to regain control of your life and become an expert in your diabetes. Whether you have been living for years with diabetes or have only recently been diagnosed, you will find much here that is positive and helpful.

AVAILABLE AUTUMN 2007

KIDNEY FAILURE EXPLAINED £17.99

Dr Andy Stein and Janet Wild

The complete reference manual that gives you, your family and friends, the information you really want to know about managing your kidney condition. Written by two experienced medical authors, this practical handbook covers every aspect of living with kidney disease – from diagnosis, drugs and treatment, to diet, relationships and sex.

> *'This book is, without doubt, the best resource currently available for kidney patients and those who care for them.'*
> VAL SAID
> kidney transplant patient

STROKE
Answers at your fingertips £17.99

Dr Anthony Rudd, Penny Irwin and Bridget Penhale

This essential guidebook tells you all about strokes – most importantly how to recover from them.

As well as providing clear explanations of the medical processes, tests, and treatments, the book is full of practical advice, including recuperation plans. You will find it inspiring.

BEATING DEPRESSION £17.99

Dr Stefan Cembrowicz and Dr Dorcas Kingham

Depression is one of most common illnesses in the world – affecting up to one in four people at some time in their lives. *Beating Depression* shows sufferers and their families that they are not alone, and offers tried and tested techniques for overcoming depression.

> *'All you need to know about depression, presented in a clear, concise and readable way.'*
> ANN DAWSON,
> World Health Organization

HEART HEALTH
Answers at your fingertips £17.99

Dr Graham Jackson

This practical handbook, written by a leading cardiologist, answers all your questions about heart conditions. It tells you all about you and your heart; how to keep your heart healthy, or if it has been affected by heart disease – how to make it as strong as possible.

> *'Those readers who want to know more about the various treatments for heart disease will be much enlightened.'*
> DR JAMES LE FANU,
> *The Daily Telegraph*

HIGH BLOOD PRESSURE
Answers at your fingertips £14.99

Dr Tom Fahey, Professor Deirdre Murphy with Dr Julian Tudor Hart

The authors use all their years of experience as blood pressure experts to answer your questions on high blood pressure, in order to give you the information you need to bring your blood pressure down – and keep it down.

> *'Readable and comprehensive information.'*
> DR SYLVIA MCLAUGHLAN,
> Director General, The Stroke Association

PRIORITY ORDER FORM

Cut out or photocopy this form and send it (post free in the UK) to:

Class Publishing　　　　　　　　　　　**Tel: 01256 302 699**
FREEPOST 16705　　　　　　　　　　　**Fax: 01256 812 558**
Macmillan Distribution
Basingstoke RG21 6ZZ

Please send me urgently　　　　　　　　　　　　*Post included*
(*tick below*)　　　　　　　　　　　　　　　*price per copy (UK only)*

☐　**Type 2 Diabetes: Answers at your fingertips**　(ISBN 978 1 85959 176 5)　　　£17.99

☐　**Type 2 Diabetes in Adults of All Ages**　(ISBN 978 1 85959 166 6)　　　£23.99

☐　**Kidney Failure Explained**　(ISBN 978 1 85959 145 1)　　　£20.99

☐　**Stroke: Answers at your fingertips**　(ISBN 978 1 85959 113 0)　　　£20.99

☐　**Beating Depression**　(ISBN 978 1 85959 150 5)　　　£20.99

☐　**Heart Health: Answers at your fingertips**　(ISBN 978 1 85959 157 4)　　　£20.99

☐　**High Blood Pressure: Answers at your fingertips**　(ISBN 978 1 85959 090 4)　　£17.99

TOTAL _____

Easy ways to pay

Cheque: I enclose a cheque payable to Class Publishing for £ _____

Credit card: Please debit my　　Mastercard　☐ Visa　☐ Amex

Number _____　　Expiry date _____

Name _____

My address for delivery is _____

_____

Town _____　County _____　Postcode _____

Telephone number (*in case of query*) _____

Credit card billing address if different from above _____

_____

Town _____　County _____　Postcode _____

Class Publishing's guarantee: remember that if, for any reason, you are not satisfied with these books, we will refund all your money, without any questions asked. Prices and VAT rates may be altered for reasons beyond our control.

BC	9/11